Staying Human during Residency Training

THIRD EDITION

This is a concise manual designed for medical students, interns, residents, and fellows in all areas of specialization. The first two editions provided hundreds of practical tips on coping with stress, sleep deprivation, time pressures, and other issues of concern to hospital residents. This newly updated version provides guidance on career choices and financial planning, as well as suggestions for enhancing personal and professional relationships. It also discusses ethical and legal matters, state-of-the-art learning strategies, and issues pertinent to women, parents, and international and minority residents.

ALLAN D. PETERKIN is an assistant professor in the Department of Psychiatry and the Department of Community and Family Medicine, University of Toronto, and is a staff psychiatrist at Mount Sinai Hospital in Toronto. He has given workshops across Canada and the United States to residents on coping with residency training. He is the author of six books on medicine and cultural history and co-author of *Caring for Lesbian and Gay People: A Clinical Guide* (University of Toronto Press, 2003).

Staying Human during Residency Training

THIRD EDITION

Allan D. Peterkin

UNIVERSITY OF TORONTO PRESS
Toronto Buffalo London

© University of Toronto Incorporated 2004
Toronto Buffalo London
Second edition 1998
Reprinted 2000
Third edition 2004
Printed in Canada

ISBN 0-8020-8615-2

Printed on acid-free paper

National Library of Canada Cataloguing in Publication

Peterkin, Allan D.
Staying human during residency training / Allan D. Peterkin. – 3rd ed.

Includes bibliographical references and index.
ISBN 0-8020-8615-2

1. Residents (Medicine) – Handbooks, manuals, etc.   I. Title.

R840.P48 2004   610'.71'55   C2003-904710-5

University of Toronto Press acknowledges the financial assistance to its publishing program of the Canada Council for the Arts and the Ontario Arts Council.

University of Toronto Press acknowledges the financial support for its publishing activities of the Government of Canada through the Book Publishing Industry Development Program (BPIDP).

For Dr Edith K. Peterkin,
my aunt, mentor, and friend

Nothing will sustain you more potently than the power to recognize in your humdrum routine, as perhaps it may be thought, the true poetry of life – the poetry of the commonplace, of the ordinary man, of the plain, toil-worn woman, with their loves and their joys, their sorrows and their griefs. The comedy, too, of life will be spread before you, and nobody laughs more often than the doctor at the pranks Puck plays upon the Titanias and the Bottoms among his patients. The humorous side is really almost as frequently turned towards him as the tragic. Lift up one hand to heaven and thank your stars if they have given you the proper sense to enable you to appreciate the inconceivably droll situations in which we catch our fellow creatures. Unhappily, this is one of the free gifts of the gods, unevenly distributed, not bestowed on all, or on all in equal proportions. In undue measure it is not without risk, and in any case in the doctor it is better appreciated by the eye than expressed on the tongue. Hilarity and good humour, a breezy cheerfulness, a nature 'sloping toward the sunny side,' as Lowell has it, help enormously both in the study and in the practice of medicine. To many of a sombre and sour disposition it is hard to maintain good spirits amid the trials and tribulations of the day, and yet it is an unpardonable mistake to go about among patients with a long face.

– Sir William Osler, The student life.
In *Aequanimitas with Other Addresses*, 3rd ed., Blakiston, New York, 1953: 397–423

Contents

Preface to the Third Edition

I began writing the first edition of *Staying Human during Residency Training* in my last year of a combined residency in psychiatry and family medicine at McGill University. By then, I had served for four years as a representative on resident issues to the Canadian Medical Association. Initially I was prompted to write this book by my own experiences of fatigue, stress, and intermittent disillusionment during training and by my observation of what had happened to some of my colleagues. On the day I wrote the preface to the first edition, I heard of a resident who by chance had left call early and found her husband walking out the door with packed bags. I had already witnessed three divorces, one psychotic break, three cases of depression needing treatment, as well as catastrophic illness among my friends and classmates. As I was preparing the second edition, one close friend was forced to do obstetrics call two days after her own miscarriage. That year my own medical school reported the suicides of three residents.

I reviewed the international literature, new and old, on stress during residency and found statistics that confirm the high-risk status of residents for drug abuse, divorce, career dissatisfaction, depression, and suicide. I saw that though many states and provinces have passed legislation to limit residents' working hours, many have not; in fact, most interns and residents in the United States still work under no formal collective agreement. I set out to write a book for residents everywhere that provides practical tips on survival (e.g., stress control, improved sleep, diet, and fitness) and information about protecting quality of life, about relationships both in and outside of medicine, and about finding a sense of joy and accomplishment in being apprentice physicians.

This third edition reflects new and emerging realities for residents across North America. It contains over 1,000 references, resources, and websites emphasizing learning, self-care, vocational guidance, and the art of healing. I believe we should thrive, not just survive, during our training.

Staying Human during Residency Training was initially written by a resident, for residents. Now, in my role as clinical professor I am reminded daily that how we teach and support each other determines, perhaps more than anything else, the kind of healers we become.

Special thanks are due to Mark Levy of CIR and Dr Laura Musselman of the CAIR Resident Wellbeing Committee for helpful suggestions in updating this new edition. Thanks also to the many medical students, residents, and fellows who have written to me and taught me so much over the years.

ALLAN D. PETERKIN, MD, CCFP, FRCP(C)
Toronto, 2003

An Appeal to Educators

This book emphasizes residents' roles in ensuring their own well-being. This focus alone is incomplete. For young physicians to stay fully human during residency training, changes must be implemented voluntarily and in good faith at the administrative and supervisory levels. The following summary of strategies for reducing residency stress at the hospital, department, and program levels is taken from 'The ravelled sleeve of care: managing the stresses of residency training,' a classic review article on residency training in the United States.

STRATEGIES TO REDUCE RESIDENCY STRESS

By Hospitals

To ensure adequate ancillary help:

- paraprofessional support (phlebotomists, electrocardiogram technicians, etc.)
- administrative support (ward clerks, messenger services, etc.)

To ensure adequate benefits:

- increased salaries
- expanded fringe benefits (medical, health, and disability insurance)
- other services (financial, legal, and tax counselling; child care and housing subsidies)

By Departments

Structural:

- 'short-stay' admissions

- grievance procedures
- physicians' extenders

Educational:

- increased faculty availability
- part-time positions ·
- formal career counselling
- 'protected time'
- management counselling

By Residency Programs

Structural:

- 'night floats'
- reduced call frequency
- redistribution of primary patient care during residency
- elimination of clinical responsibilities after nights on call
- establishment of back-up coverage for sick residents

Educational:

- training in teaching and leadership skills
- periodic feedback on performance
- training in stress-reduction methods

Morale:

- support groups for residents and spouses
- retreats
- thorough orientation for interns
- regular social events (e.g., journal clubs)
- alumni reunions with current residents

Reprinted, with permission, from Colford JM, McPhee SJ: The ravelled sleeve of care: managing the stresses of residency training. *JAMA* 1989; 261: 889–893

Staying Human during Residency Training

1. The Risks of Residency Training

Residency training can be stressful, but it also provides many opportunities for great personal and professional development. Interns and residents are not fragile; they are bright, competitive, and dedicated men and women who are eager to learn. Along with medical students, they make up approximately one-fifth of the physicians workforce, in the United States and Canada. It is striking, however, that some of the character traits that lead many people towards a career in medicine are also predictors of eventual impairment.[1]

High levels of responsibility, intense contact with people, time restrictions, role uncertainty and transition (i.e., from student to neophyte professional), sleep deprivation and social isolation are linked to distress in any profession and are all prominent in postgraduate medical education. Residents must in addition deal directly with suffering, sexuality, fear, death, uncertainty, and problem patients and staff.[2] In these circumstances, it is not surprising that they suffer varying degrees of stress-related symptoms, however healthy they may be on entering residency.

RISKS OF ANXIETY AND DEPRESSION

- In one study, 40 per cent of residents reported impaired performance as a result of anxiety or depression lasting four weeks or longer.[3]
- In another study, 29 per cent of first-year residents, 22 per cent of second-year students, and 10 per cent of third-year residents were significantly depressed.[4,5]

- In one sample, 30 per cent of residents suffered significant depression (with higher risk in the first two months of training and with work weeks of over 100 hours).[6]
- Of internal-medicine residents, 35 per cent reported four or five depressive symptoms during residency.[7]
- Almost twice the number of first-year residents (30%) are depressed compared to the general population (17%), and one in two female residents report severe depression (data presented by Dr Laura Musselman at the 2002 International Conference on Physical Health, Vancouver).

SUBSTANCE ABUSE

- In one study, 26 per cent of residents worried about drug abuse in peers, with 12 per cent reporting increased personal use of alcohol, cocaine, or marijuana, and 7 per cent increased use of sedatives.[8]
- In one sample, 11 per cent of residents used tranquillizers, and 9 per cent opiates.[8]
- Among practising physicians, 1.5 per cent are drug abusers, and 8 per cent will become dependent on alcohol.[9]

ABUSE

- 46.4–96.5 per cent of medical trainees experienced some form of abuse (verbal/sexual/physical) during their training.[10]
- In a sample of 599 female doctors, 77 per cent reported being sexually harassed by patients at least once since becoming physicians. Harassers were male in 92 per cent of cases.[11]
- Two-thirds of emergency residents worry about their own safety while working shifts.[12]

SUICIDE

- Of a resident sample taking a leave of absence, 5 per cent did so for attempted suicide.[13]
- Of a sample of depressed residentsm 25 per cent had suicidal ideation, and 18 per cent had a plan.[6]

- Physicians under forty years of age have three times the suicide risk of the general population. Suicide is the second-greatest cause of death in medical students.[14]

RELATIONSHIPS

- In two studies, 37 to 40 per cent of residents reported problems with their spouse or lover.[6,15]
- Of 1805 residents and interns, 59 per cent believed that 'role conflict was always or often a problem, in that work interfered with their family and social lives' (PAIRO Study, 1985).
- Of pediatric housestaff, 83 per cent reported experiencing stress over balancing work and family.[16]

JOB SATISFACTION

- Of residents who were asked if they would 'do it all again,' 25 per cent were not sure that they would train to be physicians (personal communication).
- In one sample, 15 per cent of residents would not repeat internship.[6]
- In a survey of Canadian medical graduates, 20 per cent would consider changing their residency discipline if possible.[17]
- Of doctors under forty surveyed by the AMA, 31 per cent would not have gone to medical school if they 'had known then what they know now.'[18]
- Doubt about specialty choice was linked to depressive symptoms.[19]

OTHER STRESSES

- Training hospitals are being sold, closed, or amalgamated.
- The average resident's salary works out to be less than U.S.$5.00 per hour.
- The debt load for Canadian residents after training is $30,000 to $100,000.
- In 1981 the average debt load after residency was U.S.$32,000 to $40,000.[21] It is now estimated to be U.S.$80,000 to $180,000.

- The average work week for Canadian and U.S. interns ranges from 90 to 120 hours, and for residents from 50 to 120 more hours in first than in second year.[22] From 20 to 22 per cent of residents work more than 80 hours per week, which is the recommended maximum. (See www.webcom.com/pgi/stress.html)
- Of a sample of internal medicine residents, 23 per cent reported becoming less humanistic, and 61 per cent more cynical during their training.[7]
- Of graduating residents, 10 per cent feel unprepared for certain clinical challenges like HIV care, substance abuse, domestic violence, and geriatrics.[23]
- Of internal medicine residents surveyed at 415 U.S. training centres, 52 per cent had insufficent funds to buy books and equipment, and 29 per cent could not afford the fees for their qualifying exams.[7]

OTHER HEALTH RISKS

- Infectious: hepatitis A, B, C; tuberculosis; Epstein-Barr virus; HIV (human immunodeficiency virus); upper respiratory tract infections; gastroenteritis; and conjunctivitis
- Chemical: radiation, anaesthetic agents, anti-neoplastic agents, and agents used in pathology laboratories (e.g., formaldehyde)
- Physical: musculoskeletal stress related to lifting and prolonged standing, violence from patients presenting to emergency departments, and lack of security in hospitals located in dangerous areas
- Women who become pregnant during residency have an increased incidence of preterm labour and pre-eclampsia.[24]

The first year of postgraduate training, especially the first two months, and rotations in medicine, surgery, and intensive care units are frequently reported to be particularly stressful. Stress-related symptoms are ubiquitous and intermittent, even when they do not become severe enough to lead to depression or drug abuse. Such symptoms can, however, lead to professional burnout, which is characterized by emotional exhaustion, depersonalization, and a low sense of accomplishment and job satisfaction.[18] Burnout is a deteriorating or unsuccessful response to repeated stress and is characterized by negative attitudes towards self, others, and work; emotional exhaustion; and feelings of despair. Other authors have referred to 'training toxicity' as being the cause of such distress.[25]

MAJOR MANIFESTATIONS OF BURNOUT[26]

Physiological

Fatigue and chronic exhaustion, persistent viral infections, headaches, lack of concentration, somatic problems, muscular pain and tension, weight problems, gastrointestinal disorders, and injuries caused by high-risk behaviour

Psychological and Emotional

Despair, feelings of impotence, disillusionment, boredom, anxiety, decreased self-esteem, guilt, mistrust, isolation from friends and family, irritability, dissatisfaction, frustration, chronic anger, memory loss, confusion, discouragement, pessimism, cynicism, and such defence mechanisms as blaming others, rationalization, displacement, and projection (*Note*: clinical major depression must be ruled out.)

Behavioural

Chronic complaining, distancing from patients' emotional needs, preoccupation with money rather than good patient care, over-prescribing of medications, absenteeism, drug addiction, impatience, inflexibility, decreased creativity and initiative, problems in interpersonal relationships, frequent shifts in mood, superficial patient contacts, non-productive hyperactivity, excessive reactions to stress, inappropriate comments, frustration, indifference, withdrawal, isolation and increased risk-taking at work

---

and in recreation, excessive criticism or devaluing of colleagues, change in consultation patterns (up or down), decreased attention to chart documentation

Organizational

Decline in quality of services, climate of hostility, competition, mistrust, authority conflicts, impaired communication, tendency to decision making in isolation, and increased sick leave, staff turnover rates

Some residents experience these symptoms only during a particularly difficult rotation, whereas others experience full-blown burnout and what has been called the 'house officer stress syndrome,' which is characterized by family problems, cynical attitudes, emotional lability and anger, personal conflict, and transient cognitive impairment.[27] A recenty study of internal medicine residents using the Maslach Burnout Inventory showed that 76 per cent of respondents met the criteria for burnout.[28] Apart from somatic and emotional symptoms, high levels of chronic malaise in young physicians can produce a lasting change of attitude towards both the medical field and patients. Residency should be a time for learning coping patterns for an active, demanding medical career, and for attaining new levels of compassion. Instead, many graduates emerge as insensitive, distant, cynical, and authoritarian physicians who make inappropriate comments and judgments about their patients. They become emotionally withdrawn and self-important, often under the guise of dedication, and their self-esteem becomes intrinsically linked to professional and financial performance, to the neglect of satisfying personal relationships.

Psychological defence mechanisms of denial and rationalization about failures, errors, and limitations; depreciation (ironic humour); isolation of affect (emotional numbness); and projection of negative feelings onto others – all of these become prominent. Many residents believe that they don't learn to communicate effectively with patients during their training, so burdened are they by technology, medical jargon, and the safe anonymity of group work and laboratory result 'rounding.' Time pressures, fatigue, and self-confidence tend to be the focus of the most difficult or stressful aspects of residency training.[22]

THE 'TOP TEN' STRESSORS[29]

1. Insufficient sleep (less than three hours)
2. Frequent night calls (every third night or more often)
3. Uncompromising attending physicians
4. Large patient load
5. Too much 'scut' work
6. Too much medical records work
7. High rates of death among patients
8. Little or no contact with fellow residents
9. Inadequate sexual activity
10. High peer competition to impress staff

Other sources of anxiety include role ambiguity with expectations beyond one's level of expertise, ethical dilemmas, information and technology overload, frequent service rotations, lack of role models, fear of lawsuits, job concerns (e.g., fear of acquiring HIV infection), and conflicts in personal and professional relationships.

The literature on resident impairment allows some degree of prediction about who is at risk in the face of high stress levels. A recent editorial in the *Annals of Internal Medicine* even posed the question, Who is sicker: patients or residents?[30] In one sample of residents, 31 per cent reported a family history of involvement with a mental health profession (Kirby Hsu). Residents who overidentify with patients and have passive-aggressive, avoidant, or dependent coping styles are predisposed to burnout. Hostile or aggressive 'Type A' residents may alienate colleagues. Those who lack support from colleagues, friends, and family exhibit more symptoms of somatic and psychological origin, and are more detached and avoidant.[31] Trainees who can't delegate responsibility or share teamwork also become more stressed.[31] Most residents experience feelings of loss of control over their lives, and even over decisions about patient care; those who report an 'external locus of control' also have higher stress levels.[32]

Most residents are twenty-five to thirty-five years old. In the most frequently studied groups (in psychiatry, internal, and family medicine programs), those in their early twenties and late thirties seem to be more affected by the rigours of residency.[33] In one study of residents in psychiatry, women and transfer students were similarly affected.[34] An Ontario study showed that women housestaff experienced more self-doubt and feelings of professional inadequacy, family practice residents worried most about making mistakes in treatment and diagnosis, and residents in psychiatry were most concerned about chronically ill patients. On-call anxiety was more frequent among residents in family medicine, psychiatry, and pediatrics. The particular challenges experienced by specific resident groups (women, international medical graduates, etc.) will be discussed in chapter 6.

The professional stresses of residency may adversely affect or postpone personal-developmental milestones because of lack of time to reflect and explore creatively. Young physicians in their twenties and thirties customarily leave their families and home towns, experience shifts in financial status, date, form sexual relationships, marry or cohabit, and have children. Some divorce, become ill, or experience a loss in their families. They search for a balance between work and play and develop interests in political and community causes. One study, which ranked developmental stressors in 243 residents in years 1 to 6 of training, found significant differences from year to year.[35] Residents in their final year, for instance, were most concerned about job prospects, and a greater proportion of residents in the first postgraduate year (than in any other year) experienced major moves and married.

The formation of a sound professional or work identity as a physician cannot be achieved independently of other developmental concerns, although the latter are often ignored. Young physicians must be able to find a balance between their own vulnerability and their role as 'non-omnipotent' healers.[36] They must recognize when to act and when to wait, observe, and listen. Residents frequently feel helpless and exploited in the medical hierarchy, but they must develop problem-solving skills that allow feelings of commitment to develop with a regained sense of personal control. They must learn 'boundary maintenance,' combining empathy with objectivity and avoiding both undue familiarity and aloofness with colleagues and patients. Residents should acquire these skills and insights as well as technical proficiency during residency training.

The emerging healer must develop a sense of identity, balance, and well-being in the face of professional and developmental stresses. The potential risks to both physical and emotional health are significant, but so are the opportunities to learn coping skills that will last throughout one's medical career. As later chapters will confirm, to be forewarned is

Figure 1.1 Stress and Coping Model for Physicians[20]

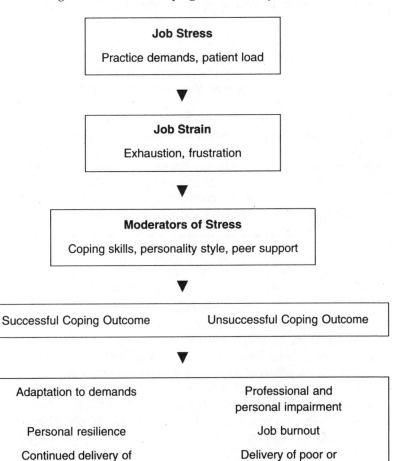

indeed to be forearmed. A coping model initially described for primary care physicians (fig. 1.1) can also be applied to all physicians and to residents in training.

The following list of elements of well-being will serve as a reference for the rest of this book and during various phases of residency itself.

NECESSARY ELEMENTS OF A PHYSICIAN'S WELL-BEING[37,38] (see chapter 3)

- Quality care, including continuity of care
- Commitment to professional values and professional growth
- Shared responsibility with the patient for the patient's health and well-being
- Full expression of the physician as an autonomous person
- Maintenance of personal physical and mental health
- Self-validation
- Recognition and acceptance of time and technological limitation, of change as a normal phenomenon, and of the profession's inherent problems and opportunities
- collegiality / work group loyalty

REFERENCES

1 Graduate medical education, Appendix II, Table 1. *JAMA* 1996; 276: 739–748; CAPER annual census of post-M.D. trainees, 1996–1997. Association of Canadian Medical Colleges, Ottawa, 1997; Blachly PH, Osterud HT, Josslin R et al: Suicide in professional groups. *N Engl J Med* 1963; 268: 1278–1282

2 McCue JD: The effects of stress on physicians and their medical practice. *N Engl J Med* 1982; 306: 458–463

3 Koran L, Litt I: House staff well-being. *West J Med* 1988; 148: 97–401

4 Reuben D: Depressive symptoms in medical house officers: effects of level of training and work rotation. *Arch Intern Med* 1985; 145: 286–288

5 Idem: Psychologic effects of residency. *South Med J* 1983; 76: 380–383

6 Valko R, Clayton P: Depression in the internship. *Dis Nerv Syst* 1975; 36: 26–269

7 Collier VU, McCue JD, Markus A, Smith L: Stress in medical residency: status quo after a decade of reform? *Ann Intern Med* 2002; 136(5): 384–395

8 McAuliffe WE, Rohmann M, Santangelo S et al: Psychoactive drug use among practicing physicians and medical students. *N Engl J Med* 1986; 315: 805–810

9 Loes M, Scheiber S: The impaired resident. *Ariz Med* 1981; 38: 777–779

10 Silver HK, Slicken, A: Medical student abuse: incidence, severity and significance. *JAMA* 1990; 263: 527–532

11 Phillips, SP: Harassment of female doctors by patients. *N Engl J Med* 1993; 329: 1936–1939

12 Anglin, D: Residents' perspectives on violence and personal safety in the emergency department. *Ann Emerg Med* 1994; 23: 1082–1084

13 Smith JW, Benny WF, Witzke DB: Emotional impairment in internal medicine house staff. *JAMA* 1979; 255: 1155–1158

14 Ross M: Suicide among physicians. *Psychiatry Med* 1971; 2: 189–198

15 Landau C, Hall S, Wartman SA et al: Stress in social and family relationships during medical residency. *J Med Educ* 1986; 61: 654–660

16 Kahn JA, Parsons SK, Pizzo PA, Newburger JW, Homer CJ: Work-family issues and perceptions of stress among pediatric faculty and house staff. *Ambul Pediatr* 2001; 1(3): 141–149

17 Rafuse J: Negative health care environment weighing on residents: survey. *J Can Med Assoc* 1997; 156(8): 118

18 Reported in *Globe and Mail Report on Business*. June 1994

19 Hainer BL, Palesch Y: Symptoms of depression in residents: a South Carolina Family Practice Research Consortium study. *Acad Med* 1998; 73(12): 1305–1310

20 May HH, Revicki DA: Professional stress among family physicians. *J Fam Pract* 1985; 20: 165–171

21 Rudner HL: Stress and coping mechanisms in a group of family practice residents. *J Med Educ* 1985; 60: 564–566

22 Idem: Stress in family practice residents. *Can Fam Physician* 1986; 32: 319–323

23 Greene, I. *AMNews* (24 Sept 01, online)

24 Klebanoff, MA: Outcomes of pregnancy in a national sample of resident physicians. *N Engl J Med* 1990; 323: 1040–1045.

25 Carius, M: Avoiding training toxicity. *Annals of Emerg Med* 2001; 38(5): 596–597.

26 Bouchard F, Bélanger P (eds): *Putting the Heat on Burnout, Health and Safety.* Committee of the Fédération des infirmières et imfirmiers de Québec, Litho Acme, Quebec, 1989

27 Small GW: House officer stress syndrome. *Psychosom Med* 1981; 22: 860–869

28 Shanafelt TD, Bradley KA, Wipf JE, Back AL: Burnout and self-reported patient care in an internal medicine residency program. *Ann Intern Med* 2002; 136(5): 358–367

29 Schwartz AJ, Black ER, Goldstein MG: Levels and causes of stress among residents. *J Med Educ* 1987; 62: 744–753

30 Hawes, L: Who is sicker: patients or residents? Residents' distress and the care of patients. *Ann Intern Med* 2002; 136(5): 391–393

31 Mazie B: Job stress, psychological health, and social support of family practice residents. *J Med Educ* 1985; 60: 935–941

32 Frey J, Demick J, Bibace R: Variations in physicians' feelings of control during a family practice residency. *J Med Educ* 1981; 56: 50–56

33 Rudner HL: Work-related stress: a survey of family practice residents in Ontario. *Can Fam Physician* 1988; 34: 577–583

34 Russell AT, Pasnace RO, Taintor ZC: Emotional problems of residents in psychiatry. *Am J. Psychiatry* 1975; 132: 263–267

35 Taylor AD, Sinclair A, Wall EM: Sources of stress in postgraduate medical training. *J Med Educ* 1987; 62: 425–428

36 Brent DA: The residency as a developmental process. *J Med Educ* 1981; 56: 417–422

37 Garell DC: Some reflections on physicians' well being. *New Physician* 1978; 27: 32–33 (chart adapted with permission)

38 Randall CS, Bergus GR, Schlechte JA, McGuinness G, Mueller CW: Factors associated with primary care residents' satisfaction with their training. *Fam Med* 1997; 29(10): 730–735

OTHER SOURCES

Gatrell J, White T: *The Specialist Registrar Handbook*. Radcliffe Medical Press, Abingdon, Eng., 1999
Oxon (covers training issues in the United Kingdom)
Posen, David B: Stress management for patient and physician. *Can J CME* April 1995; 45–50

2. *Choosing a Humane Residency*

Until fairly recently, graduating medical students, when choosing a residency program, focused more on the program's reputed standards or prestige than on the quality of life they could expect during that four- to six-year period of their lives. They sometimes based their choices on hearsay or information acquired by chance. In interviews they concentrated on practical questions such as the size of a program or the opportunities it offered for research. Because selection was highly competitive, students seldom introduced other, more human concerns for fear of appearing demanding or not sufficiently dedicated.

Three trends in North America seem to have produced a change in the attitudes of candidates and residency directors towards such concerns. First, the growing number of women in medicine, who now constitute about 40 to 50 per cent of most U.S. and Canadian medical classes, has forced universities to consider part-time and shared residencies as well as parental leaves. Such modifications in response to women's demands have been achieved with great struggle; yet men now acknowledge that they also benefit from these new policies.[1]

Second, restrictions on the number of hours worked by interns and residents have started to increase in reaction to lawsuits (such as the well-publicized Libby Zion case in New York) stemming from errors made by overworked and undersupervised interns.

A final trend stems from the drop in demand for entry to undergraduate medical classes in the United States.[2] Currently numbers are down 26 per cent from 1996 to 35,000 in 2002, with a 33 per cent decrease in male applications. With fewer than two applicants for each first-year place, many residency programs are becoming concerned about filling positions. Some will gradually increase the workload for the residents they do have; others will respond by competing to attract graduating medical students to achieve their quotas. In some ways, then, residency training programs might become potentially more sensitive to residents' growth and comfort than was the case ten years ago. On the other hand, managed care, with its emphasis on cost-effectiveness, has seen the closing of hundreds of residency slots in many U.S. programs.[2] As well, some students have reported that navigating the National Resident Matching Program (NRMP) has become more complicated and prone to violations.[2] Overall, the choice of program has become more complicated because more factors now influence the selection of a specialty.

PROGRAM FACTORS

Because of the considerable variation in the size, content, and administration of residency programs across the United States and Canada, medical graduates must exercise great care in their choice of program to try to ensure maximum learning and personal satisfaction.[3] This means gathering a large body of information about each centre from a variety of sources before applying, because it is not possible to discover accurately all the features of a program in a single interview.

Data should be obtained from the program or hospital prospectus, medical school counsellors, published specialty manuals such as the American Psychiatric Association's Directory of Psychiatric Residency Training Programs (for psychiatry),[4] the Fellowship and Residency Electronic Interactive Database (FREIDA), the National Resident Matching Program Handbook for Students (see resources), local faculty members at the undergraduate and postgraduate levels, and student members of specialty associations.

Classmates gathering similar data can share facts and ideas. It is a good idea to make informal contact with junior and senior residents at each centre being considered, or perhaps with graduates of one's own school, and to obtain a copy of the hospital, state, or provincial contract for residents. A day-long visit to the teaching hospital can help one assess working conditions and resident morale. Applicants should ensure that they have gathered all pertinent information before accepting a residency position.

CONSIDERATIONS IN CHOOSING A RESIDENCY[5]

The Program

- number of residents in each year of the program and the number expected to begin in the first year of the next session
- number of hospitals in the program
- amount of time spent in each hospital
- financial resources of the program
- location of each hospital
- amount, location, and flexibility in scheduling and content of elective time
- amount of supervision, volume of activity, and length of shifts in emergency rotations
- anticipated major shifts in program policy or administration that might affect residents
- availability of rural/primary care rotations and clinical exposure
- cost of living in specific urban centre
- potential for advancement (fellowships, chief residency, and staff positions)
- success rate of residents in fellowship or board exams
- availability of support groups and resources (see chapter 4)
- resident satisfaction/input to program design

The Specialty

- spousal preference regarding lifestyle/location
- lifestyle and workload
- job and academic prospects
- competitiveness and availability of programs
- expected salary and medical school debt load
- lawsuit potential
- sexual stereotyping
- age preference (young versus old patients)
- length of training
- balance between emphasis on patient contact and communication skills and on manual and technical skills
- research potential, scientific interests

- local licensing requirements ('portability' of the specialty)
- personal issues (family or personal history of a particular illness)
- success and satisfaction levels in undergraduate rotations
- positive exposure to resident or mentor role models
- family factors (family member in the same specialty, partner's preferences)
- intellectual preference and background
- availability of subspecialty options
- personality style
- public and media perceptions of the specialty
- perceived personal health risk (burnout, infectious diseases)
- government manpower 'shortage' policies (incentives/disincentives) affecting practice-setting options on graduation
- autonomy versus team approach

The Institution

- unionized or non-unionized; availability of resident representation
- type (specialized, military, private, county, provincial or state)
- availability of resources and innovative techniques
- number of beds and admissions per year
- research and teaching possibilities
- popularity of the hospital among housestaff
- commitment to teaching versus service
- involvement of HMOs / managed care and how that affects exposure to a broad clinical base and continuity of care
- patient type (geographic area served, socio-economic and ethnic status, variety in age, and proportion of acute versus chronic problems)

Attending Staff

- background of the service chief and attending staff
- availability of the residency training director
- interest and availability of staff for teaching, consulting, supervising, and mentoring
- exposure to well-known clinicians in field

> **Duties**
>
> - time spent on service versus teaching
> - expected ward patient load
> - organization of rotations: emergency, elective, chronic, clinic, and inpatient
> - frequency of night calls, number of residents on call and extent of cross-coverage of wards
> - scheduling of rounds (mornings, weekends, etc.)
> - expectations regarding follow-up on patients treated on wards or in emergency department
> - 'scut' level and availability of support staff: nurses, physicians' assistants/extenders, paramedics, blood and intravenous drip teams, messengers, porters, librarians, secretarial staff, and medical records staff
> - legislated limits to number of hours worked / contract protec- . tions

THE HUMAN FACTOR

Learning and training considerations should always be balanced against those that affect quality of life. Residents pay rent, manage debts, go on holiday, have social commitments, and perhaps raise a family; therefore, they need financial information on salary level, frequency of payment (weekly or biweekly), and possibly moonlighting. Benefits such as life, health, disability, and malpractice insurance should be provided or made available at reasonable rates through the hospital housestaff union or local medical association.

Applicants may want to know about policies and practices on maternity or paternity leave, job sharing, part-time residency, and compassionate and sick leave. The size of the program will determine the level of familiarity and intimacy among staff, residents, and patients. Some may view residency as a time to explore new approaches in a new city; others may decide to settle where they have completed medical school so as to build a reputation and career there.

Applicants also need to learn about the availability, cost, and safety of housing, and about its proximity to the hospital. They may want to know whether schools, day care, and shopping facilities are nearby. A support system of family and friends provides protection against stress during residency, and its presence or absence may affect the decision to relocate. Climate and cultural events or athletic facilities may also be important considerations.

Many residents believe that raising such matters during an interview may jeopardize their chances of acceptance because they may introduce personal information – about marital status, plans to have children, health, and so on – that may not be supplied otherwise. It may be wise to obtain information about these issues elsewhere, but a program that penalizes an applicant for raising them, or that has no provision for such benefits or resources, may not be desirable.

This personal and professional information must be sorted out if applicants are to choose a program where they will learn happily. Family members, medical school counsellors or mentors, friends, and significant others should all be recruited to help weigh the elements involved.

THE INTERVIEW

This is your chance to determine if a program is right for you. Dress professionally and comfortably, and pay attention to grooming. Arm yourself with as much information as possible about a program before your interview. You can then be attentive to important details that will help you make your final decision. Was the program helpful and flexible in making arrangements to meet you? Are interviewers punctual? Do they put you at ease? (One resident in psychiatry reported that an interviewer in Chicago asked him to leave the room and return as his mother!) Know and note the names and titles/positions of all interviewers and consider sending them a follow-up thank-you note. Be courteous to all support staff you contact around the interviews, as they may be asked their opinion of you. Certain topics and questions should not be raised by interviewers in Canada and the United States because they are inappropriate on human rights grounds. You should nevertheless prepare for them because they invariably arise.

Inappropriate Interview Questions

- How old are you?
- What is your marital status?
- What is your sexual orientation?
- Do you have plans for marriage or pregnancy?
- Outline your medical and psychiatric history.
- What is your HIV sero-status?

- What is your ethnic and family background?
- Will you select the program if you are ranked highly? (This violates Match agreements, though you may wish to volunteer this information. Don't rely on verbal promises.)
- Where else have you interviewed?

Asking 'May I know why you ask that?' in response to such questions suggests to the interviewer that certain details are private and gives you time to compose a suitable response.

Some provocative questions are reasonable and appropriate. You should not only expect them but also rehearse your replies, because they will give an interviewer an accurate sense of your character and career goals. Be sure to appear interested, motivated, and enthusiastic.

Expected Interview Questions

- Tell me about yourself. What makes you unique?
- What are your weaknesses and strengths?
- What are your long-term plans?
- Is there anything about you that might prevent you from successfully completing your residency in 'x' years?
- What is your most important achievement to date?
- Why have you selected 'x' as a specialty? Why not 'y'?
- What is the most significant error you have made in your clinical work so far? How did you correct it?
- What attracted you to this program?
- What are your interests outside of medicine?
- Have you any questions about our program?
- Have you any plans to do research or teach?
- How are you at teamwork?
- Where do you plan to be ten years from now?
- What do you want out of life?
- Tell me about a significant medical error you witnessed and how you dealt with it.
- Tell me about 'x' (a recent news event or recent medical breakthrough).
- What have you been reading outside of medicine lately?

BEFORE SIGNING ON: WHAT TO LOOK FOR IN RESIDENCY CONTRACTS[6,7]

The AMA has published a document called 'Guidelines for Housestaff Contracts or Agreements.' CAIR (the Canadian Association of Interns and Residents) and CIR (the Committee of Interns and Residents, in the United States) can also be contacted for contractual questions. (See the Resources section at the end of this book.)

Among the essential points to look for in a written agreement are:

- specified salary year by year (which should be the same for all residents at your level)
- work hours (including maximum call and days off)
- available leave (including bereavement, illness, personal/family, educational – with duration specified)
- no limitations on off-duty involvements (i.e., you're free to moonlight)
- contract termination procedures and appeal possibilities (related to quitting, transferring, or being fired)
- transfer provisions (should your program close or amalgamate)
- other benefits (living quarters, uniforms/laundry, meals, staff health services, pagers, lockers, library facilities)
- policies related to sexual harassment, discrimination, disciplinary protocols, and grievances
- flexibility regarding changing programs

(Adapted from New guidelines for resident contracts, *JAMA* 1996; 276(1): 26)

PREPARING A CURRICULUM VITAE

Type clearly on quality white 8½ x 11 inch paper.

1. Name
2. Permanent address
3. Phone number
4. Languages (optional)
5. Medical education (name of school and year of graduation; G.P.A./ class ranking are optional)
6. Postgraduate and postsecondary education (degrees earned, years, school, location; undergraduate education; high school; military experience)
7. Scholarships and prizes (list in reverse chronological order, most recent first)
8. Publications and presentations (in reverse order, most recent first)
9. Employment, research, and summer activities (in reverse order; emphasize long-term positions and medically related fields)

10   Special academic/research interests
11. Current society organizations/clubs/memberships
12. Hobbies and interests/career goals
13. Personal data (*Note*: Details such as race, marital status, children, and citizenship are *optional*. Include them only if you wish to be asked)
14. References (include names, titles, addresses, and phone numbers)
15. Date of CV (i.e., Fall 2004)

Note: A photo, date of birth, and social insurance number may be requested by the program.

REFERENCES

1 Gray K: Critical condition. *Details*, Sept 2002: 149
2 Mattix H: Managed care and residency training. *JAMA* 1996; 276(13): 1087
3 Carek PJ: Residency selection process and the match: does anybody believe anybody? *JAMA* 2001; 285(21): 2784–2785
4 Robinowitz CB et al: *Directory of Psychiatry Residency Training Programs*, 5th ed. Am Psychiatric Assoc, Washington, DC, 1997
5 Raff MJ, Schwartz IS: An applicant's evaluation of a medical house officership. *N Engl J Med* 1974; 293: 601–605
6 New guidelines for resident contracts. *JAMA* 1996; 276: 26
7 Wischnitzer S: *Survival Guide for Medical Students*. Hanely and Belfus, Philadelphia, 2001

ADDITIONAL READING/RESOURCES

AMA-FREIDA website: www.ama-assn.org/freida. Check out the 'Resources for Residents' section of the AMA website (ama-assn.org) for regularly updated content on navigating the match, transitioning in residency, contract information, preparing a CV, resident work hours policies, and student loan debt relief.
AMSA's Student Guide to Appraisal and Selection of Housestaff Training Programs. AMSA, Reston, Virginia, 1990
Annual Report on Graduate Medical Education (yearly in December issue of *JAMA*)
Canadian Resident Matching Service: carmsmai@carms.ca
Council of Teaching Hospitals Directory, American Assoc. of Medical Colleges (AAMC): published yearly

Directory of Graduate Medical Education Programs, AMA: published yearly

Electronic Residency Application Service (ERAS): www.aamc.org/eras

GMED Companion: An Insider's Guide to Selecting a Residency Program by American Medical Association, Chicago; updated annually

Iserson KV: *Getting into a Residency: A Guide for Medical Students*. Galen Press, Columbia, SC, 2000

Miller L: *Medical Students' Guide to Successful Residency Matching*. Williams and Wilkin, Lippincott, Philadelphia, 2001

National Residency Matching Program Directory (NRPM)

Peterkin A: There are some questions residency interviewers have no right to ask. *Can Med Assoc J* 1989; 140: 325

Taylor A: *How to Choose a Medical Specialty*, 3rd ed. Saunders, Philadelphia, 1999

Virtual Family Medicine Interest group: covers issues related to research, choosing a residency, arranging interviews, navigating the match, and relocating. http://fmignet.aafp.org/residency.html

3. Living, Learning, and Teaching with No Time

DIET

No one has studied the nutritional status of physicians in training or their particular needs, but several known factors suggest that they do not eat well. Stress and lack of sleep may suppress the appetite or lead to increased consumption of junk food or caffeine. Time pressure, and poor quality or variety of hospital cafeteria food, often make residents decide to skip meals entirely. The hypothalamic response to prolonged stress – such as occurs in residency – results in increased turnover of protein, carbohydrates, and fats and, if severe, may deplete vitamin and mineral reserves. This is itself a physiologic stress factor. Although nutrition guidelines now recommend a specific daily intake from each of the four food groups (dairy, meat/protein, breads/cereals, and fruits/vegetables), several modifications can be useful.

Small frequent meals fit more easily than large ones into crowded schedules, produce less postprandial fatigue, and may lessen stress-induced dyspepsia or nausea, a common complaint of housestaff. Eating foods with a high fibre content will prevent changes in bowel habits, whereas a high level of fluid intake will prevent dehydration. Healthy snacks from the hospital cafeteria and vending machines should replace chocolate, pastries, and caffeinated beverages. Sweet snacks give only short-lived energy boosts, followed by rapid swings in blood sugar levels with resultant 'crash' or 'let-down' fatigue. Caffeine may be tempting if you are tired, but it may produce increased anxiety, tremor, and diuresis.

Many of these healthy foods can be requested of the hospital and stocked in the interns' lounge or lockers so that they are available when meals are missed. Vitamin supplementation remains a controversial issue because there is no definitive proof that increased emotional stress depletes nutritional stores. A 'B-C-E-mineral' complex may, however, be useful in the face of irregular eating habits and skipped meals. Certainly a woman with a tendency towards anemia will have impaired energy levels if she does not receive an iron supplement.

FUEL-EFFICIENT SNACKS

- fruit (apples and pears)
- low-fat yogurt, cheese, skim milk (high in protein, may boost energy)
- bagels, bread, and toast (with jam)
- dried fruit (e.g., raisins)
- graham crackers and ginger snaps
- carrots and celery
- pretzels
- nuts

EATING STRATEGIES

- Eat small meals frequently.
- Have only light meals before sleep.
- Eat a diet composed of 55 per cent carbohydrates, less than 30 per cent fat, and 15 per cent protein.
- Consider vitamin supplementation.
- Decrease intake of caffeine, tobacco, alcohol, fatty foods, and simple carbohydrates.
- Increase your intake of complex carbohydrates.
- Avoid fad dieting.
- Pack snacks for on-call periods.

SUBSTANCE ABUSE

Increased levels of stress, as described in chapter 1, can provoke increased alcohol consumption and use of cigarettes and both illicit and prescription drugs. Cigarette smoking may suppress your appetite and results in increased vitamin C requirements. Alcohol binges during time off may produce a hangover with characteristic symptoms of headache, nausea, and decreased reaction time, but they also may result in dehydration and vitamin B depletion. The street drugs most often used by housestaff are stimulants (cocaine and amphetamines) and appetite suppressants, but prescription narcotics (like oxycodone) and tranquillizers (especially benzodiazepenes) are used as well.

SIGNS OF PERSONAL PROBLEMS WITH ALCOHOL OR DRUGS

- denial or secretive behaviour about use
- self-treatment, self-prescribing
- increased use of the substance, including frequent binges
- use of the substance as a crutch or coping device (e.g., to get through a stressful event)
- increased feeling of loss of control ('Who cares?')
- inability to cut back; repeated and ineffective decisions to stop using substance
- decreased functioning at work (errors, legal or financial complications, absenteeism, starting or staying late)
- family, friends, and colleagues express concern about use
- increased conflict with others owing to personality changes, mood swings, irritability
- being 'stoned' (intoxicated) at work
- health problems related to use (e.g., alcohol-related gastritis)
- tolerance to increased intake (i.e., need for greater amounts to produce the same effect)
- symptoms of emotional and physical withdrawal when attempts are made to stop

---

Drug use, abuse, and options for help are discussed in chapter 5.

SLEEP

A lack of sleep represents perhaps the most significant stress to physicians in training, who commonly work thirty-six-hour shifts as frequently as every second to every fourth day. While on duty, they average 2.7 hours of sleep. Although studies of shift workers abound,[1-4] only a few controversial ones have examined interns and residents. They have shown a variety of effects of reduced sleep and fatigue: decreased mathematical ability, less accuracy in electrocardiogram reading, memory deficit, irritability, impaired concentration, depersonalization, inappropriate affect, and decreased cognitive performance and fine motor skills. One study noted post-call car accidents in 35 per cent of a sample of medical interns who were followed up for one month.[5]

Other professions have acknowledged categorically the risks attendant on sleep deprivation. Nurses, air pilots, air traffic and other transportation controllers and operators, army recruits, and nuclear inspectors and attendants all have regulated hours for reasons of individual and corporate safety. It is acknowledged by sleep experts that at least five hours of sleep are required for a worker to maintain cognitive and motor skills.[6] Medicine has been slow to acknowledge this risk to trainees and patients, in part because of the cost of replacement services and in part because of a traditional stoicism that equates forgoing sleep with dedication. A growing number of studies, reviews, and commentaries by occupational health and legal experts are advancing compelling arguments for residency work schedule reform. They also offer strategies for implementing change.[7,8] The 2002 Sleep in America poll, for instance, revealed that if patients learned that resident surgeons were up for twenty-four hours, 86 per cent would feel anxious and 70 per cent would ask for another doctor. (For more information on this and more recent surveys, check www.sleepfoundation.org or www.amsa.org.) Other studies have demonstrated better cost and work efficiency when housestaff are less fatigued.[6] Residents with modified working schedules are likely to make fewer medication errors, increase their productivity, and discharge patients faster.

Frequently changing or disrupted sleep schedules and sleep deprivation alter natural circadian rhythms and cause gastrointestinal complaints (e.g., indigestion, constipation, and dyspepsia), anorexia, mood swings, chronic fatigue, and irritability. One study showed that up to 25 per cent of all beeper pages were unimportant or unnecessary and actually interrupted patient care.[9] People with diabetes, epilepsy, depression, and respiratory disorders are at higher medical risk when they are deprived of sleep because of disrupted physiological cycles and altered efficacy or absorption of medications that are designed to coincide with these rhythms.

THE TOP 10 COGNITIVE/NEUROBEHAVIOURAL EFFECTS
OF FATIGUE[10]

1. Alertness and vigilance become unstable; lapses of attention increase.
2. Cognitive slowing occurs; time pressure increases errors.
3. Working memory declines.
4. Tasks may be begun well, but performance deteriorates with increasing rapidity.
5. Perseveration on ineffective solutions.
6. Growing neglect of activities judged to be nonessential (loss of situational awareness).
7. Involuntary microsleep attacks occur.
8. Increased compensatory effort required to remain effective.
9. Risks of critical errors and accidents increase.
10. Cognitive deficits can be masked by stimulation.

David Dinges, PhD

Unreasonable call schedules predominate in most North American training programs today. You should therefore adopt strategies to ensure needed rest. Planning and conducting rounds before retiring, including giving clear instructions to nursing staff about pending laboratory results or vital-sign changes, can prevent unnecessary calls. Ideally you should have your own room key and ready access to a telephone and bathroom/shower, and you should have the option to stay overnight in the room if late working hours make it inconvenient or unsafe for you to return home. In addition, it is not unreasonable to ask the head nurse or nursing supervisor to screen nursing requests before you are paged. Splitting the night with a colleague (midnight to 4 a.m., 4 a.m. to 8 a.m.) can ensure four hours of sleep without frequent interruption. Call-room facilities should be quiet, cleanly maintained, close to wards, and unshared (i.e., one person to a room). Ideally, support staff should be recruited to do the 'scut' work, tasks that housestaff are usually expected to do at night. When possible, you should be paired with another resident to permit task splitting (e.g., emergency admission versus ward work), and you should be allowed to leave the next day after signing off patient care post-call.

A shift system should be carefully designed and tried. Shifts that begin at noon, 10 p.m. and 2 a.m. seem to be least disruptive of circadian rhythms, as are either rapid shift rotations (every few days) or extended numbers of days on a specific shift pattern. In June 2002, AMA delegates released a policy recommendation calling for the limiting of total residency hours to eighty per week, averaged for a two-week period, and encouraged the Accreditation Council for Graduate Medical Education (ACGME) to enforce accreditation standards regarding resident hours. Other measures suggested restricting on-call assignments to twenty-four hours, limited scheduling to one in three calls, and required one day off in seven. Check out these websites for ongoing updates regarding work hour policies in the United States: www.ama-assn.org, www.amsa.org, and www.sleepfoundation.org.

TEN TIPS FOR FIRST AND SUBSEQUENT CALL NIGHTS

1. Pay close attention at evening sign-out rounds to particular problems with patients. Prioritize the sickest patients. Make a 'scut' list. Clarify management instructions from your senior resident.
2. Clarify with your senior how to proceed during call if you have questions and how to reach him or her to discuss cases. Clarify your role with the medical student as well. Do not hesitate to ask for teaching or help – that is why you are there.
3. Make sure your beeper works. Respond to pages quickly.
4. Prevent rather than treat. When you see a patient on a ward, ask if there are other concerns/problems while you're there.
5. When you are called to assess someone, see the patient, and write a timed and dated note on every patient (as legal documentation and medical update). Leave clear instructions with the nurse about when to call you again. If the nurse calls to inform you of something, discuss whether the patient needs to be seen.
6. Carry good pocket manuals for differential diagnosis and treatment guidelines.
7. Organize your time strategically. Deal with all problems and review all laboratory and x-ray results service by service or

floor by floor. Keep a detailed list. Assessing the patient and writing orders in the emergency department will save you travel time and even 'scut' work, because most tests and bloods sampling can be done there.

8. Although you have backup and may not even be the first to see patients, discipline yourself to conduct thorough physical exams, differential diagnoses, work-ups, and treatment plans to avoid the temptation, especially when tired, to readily accept someone else's management. After residency you will not have this opportunity to test yourself under supervision.

9. Rehearse particular emergency management plans in your mind on the way to assess the patient. This will reduce anxiety and increase efficiency. *On-call Principles and Protocols* is an excellent book that takes you step by step through key on-call problems and their management.[11]

10. Determine sign-over time the next morning and your role then (e.g., presentation of new admissions). Look after yourself the next day!

TIPS FOR REGULAR SLEEP

- Aim for a consistent post-call sleeping pattern or ritual.
- Take a twenty-minute 'wind down' period or warm bath before going to bed.
- Reduce the frequency of large meals and intake of greasy foods before retiring, but eat enough to prevent your waking hungry.
- Reduce or eliminate alcohol, caffeine, and tranquillizer consumption before retiring.
- Increase exercise, but not immediately before bedtime.
- Use the bed for sleep only; if you cannot sleep, do something else out of bed and delay your usual bedtime by one or two hours.
- Use ear plugs, unplug the phone, and make sure the temperature and noise levels of you sleeping quarters are comfortable.

EXERCISE

Regular exercise seems almost impossible to schedule for most interns and residents because of fatigue and time pressure. It takes some inventiveness to incorporate exercise into a busy routine. Aerobic exercise, for periods of twenty to thirty minutes, three times a week, is an ideal solution to emotional stress because it enhances relaxation through endorphin release, decreases depressive symptoms, increases energy levels, improves sleep, dampens the fight-or-flight response, and improves the physiologic response to emotional and physical challenge. Many residents walk or run to work and climb stairs at work rather than take the elevator. Others buy an exercycle or rowing machine for home use, live in an apartment complex with a pool or sports facilities, or join a gym near the hospital. Others arrange to use facilities in the hospital such as the pool or Nautilus machines in the physiotherapy department.

Besides regular exercise, various simple techniques of relaxation can significantly reduce physical tension, anxiety, and fatigue.[12]

SIMPLE RELAXATION EXERCISES

Abdominal Breathing

Most people under stress take frequent, quick, shallow breaths using only their diaphragms. To change this pattern, use the abdomen and take deeper breaths, by letting your belly fall out. Breaking inspiration into sniffs to the count of four and then exhaling to the count of four soon induces relaxation. Each breathing cycle takes eight seconds; the appearance of sighing signals that the exercise is working.

Shoulder Shrugs

Shrugging your shoulders reduces tensions in the upper body, which is usually affected during periods of stress. Inhale while pulling your shoulders up towards your head; rotate your shoulders so that your shoulder blades come together and exhale while letting your shoulders fall back down. Three to five repetitions in a sitting or standing position usually result in quick relief.

Head Rolls

Relieve neck tension by exhaling while letting your chin fall toward your chest. Breathe in while rotating your head to the right and to the back, and then exhale while rotating your head to the left and forward to your chest. Repeat three to five cycles in a sitting or standing position.

Progressive Muscular Relaxation

This is a useful technique that can also be taught to patients who feel under stress. Alternately tense and relax each muscle group in sequence from your toes up to your buttocks; extend or puff out your abdomen and chest; finally, progressively tense and relax your fingers, arms, shoulders, and facial muscles. Do this exercise while you are lying down in a quiet place, inhaling during the muscular tension phase of a few seconds and exhaling during a few seconds of letting the muscles go limp. Five minutes should be sufficient for this total-body relaxation exercise.

PROTECTING YOUR PHYSICAL HEALTH

- Update your immunizations. Arrange for a diphtheria/tetanus (DT) booster if your last vaccination was more than ten years ago.
- Arrange for tuberculin skin testing so that you know your status and can be assessed after exposure, and followed up or treated if necessary. Inquire about hospital policy on TB enforcement. (The U.S. Center for Disease Control suggests yearly TB testing for health-care workers.)
- Arrange for measles, polio, and rubella vaccination if you have not been vaccinated or if you have no history of any of these diseases.
- Women of child-bearing age should have a rubella hemagglutination inhibition test to determine their immune status.
- Mumps vaccination is optional but is strongly advised in the absence of previous vaccination or documented disease. Influenza vaccination is also optional but is advised for those at increased risk of, for example, asthma, diabetes, severe anemia, immunodeficiency, and heart or renal disease. Discuss these vaccinations with your staff health office.

- Heptavac (Hepatitis B vaccine) given at zero, one, and six months is strongly advised and should be provided free of charge by your hospital. Both plasma-derived and recombinant forms have been proven safe and effective. Your work as a resident puts you at risk of contracting Hepatitis B; do not take the chance.
- Havrix (Hepatitis A vaccine) is also available and recommended.
- Prevent lower-back injuries by avoiding excessive leaning over a patient; raise the bed, not the patient. Pay attention to posture when you are sitting or standing for prolonged periods. Obtain help when lifting patients or equipment. Get close to the patient or object and lift with your legs. Ask an orderly to show you how.
- Avoid radiation exposure by standing at least 18 metres from portable x-ray equipment. Ask for a portable radiation meter if you are working in an area of high exposure (e.g., radiology).
- Request adequate training for the handling of toxic substances (i.e., anti-neoplastic agents) and information on local 'Right To Know' laws about exposure to toxic materials.

Protecting Yourself from Physical Violence[13,14]

DANGER SIGNS OF VIOLENCE IN A PATIENT

By History

- past history of violence/criminal involvement
- threats of violence
- poor social functioning (i.e., conflict with authority, job/school conflicts)
- history of childhood sexual/physical abuse
- personality disorders (antisocial/borderline)

By Diagnosis

- alcohol/drug intoxication or withdrawal
- acute mania/psychosis (including command hallucinations)
- organic brain syndrome/delirium
- seizures (temporal lobe, partial or complex)

Behavioural

- loud, threatening speech
- tense, clenched posture
- agitation/restlessness
- pacing, easy to startle
- rapid breathing
- violent gestures (pounding the table, pointing)

Strategies to Ensure Safety

- Familiarize yourself with security measures already in place (video cameras, alarm buzzers; weapon/firearm checks by security; hospital emergency 'code' protocols).
- Review hospital procedures for physical restraint.
- Warn others of high-risk behaviours if you witness them. Don't allow a situation to escalate.
- Watch how you dress. Accessories, ties, pens, pins, necklaces, chains, scissors are all potential weapons. Long hair can be pulled.
- Be courteous and non-provocative regardless of the patient's behaviour. Do not lecture, condescend, or express annoyance.
- Make sure the examining area is well lit and clutter-free (i.e., with no throwable objects).
- Never stand between the patient and the door, and make sure *you* have the closest access to the exit or door.
- If you feel you are in danger, do not continue the exam/interview. Leave at once and caution security.
- When in doubt about a patient, call a support staff member or request the presence of a third party.
- Do not stare at, point at, or touch an angry patient..
- If a patient is agitated, request physical restraint during your examination, especially if drawing blood.
- Be cautious leaving hospital grounds at night. If in doubt, take a taxi or request that a security guard accompany you to your car.

Avoiding Viral/Bacterial Infections

- Follow stringently all isolation and hand-washing precautions for both your safety and that of your patients. Keep your hands away from your eyes and face to reduce the incidence of viral infections.

- Reduce your risk of needle-stick injuries by *never* recapping needles; never manipulate used scalpel blades without an instrument; never leave used needles around (e.g., on beds); dispose of all sharp objects in an appropriate container that is not full; and seek help for blood-related procedures when a patient is agitated. Should you sustain a needle-stick injury, let the wound bleed, wash it with soap and water, disinfect it with alcohol, and then immediately call the staff health unit for follow-up procedures. New medical protocols for post-HIV exposure (i.e., drug therapy) now exist.
- Make sure that all equipment you use is adequately maintained, disinfected/sterilized.
- Use precautions against human immunodeficiency virus (HIV) infection.[15] Follow the universal blood and body-fluid precautions and recommendations concerning handling body fluids and procedures for using gloves and washing hands listed in the table below.

UNIVERSAL BLOOD AND BODY-FLUID PRECAUTIONS

Body fluids for which gloves followed by hand-washing are recommended:

- blood
- blood-contaminated fluids
- sperm
- cerebrospinal fluid
- pleural fluid
- pericardial fluid
- peritoneal fluid
- synovial fluid
- amniotic fluid

Body fluids for which gloves are not recommended (if not contaminated by blood), but hand-washing *is* recommended:

- saliva
- stools, diarrhoea
- vomitus
- tears

- nasal secretions
- oral secretions

Procedures for which gloves followed by hand-washing are recommended:

- intubation
- bronchoscopy
- dental procedures
- wound irrigation
- phlebotomy
- finger and/or heel stick
- vascular catheter placement
- tracheotomy suctioning
- rinsing of used instruments
- lumbar puncture
- amniocentesis
- puncture of other cavities

Note: Masks and eye barrier protection should be used *whenever* splattering is likely. Diaper changing is usually done without gloves but followed immediately by hand washing.

ILLNESS

Residents and interns are not immune from health problems, though they like to believe that they are. The following suggestions are made to residents who become ill during training.

- Do not use denial to avoid receiving the medical attention you need.
- Maintain a good link with your treating physician, who can see or refer you, or admit you to hospital quickly.
- Do not self-treat and do not play 'doctor games' with your physician about knowledge and control issues. Find someone competent and caring and let yourself be cared for; relinquish the need for total control.
- Do not expect special treatment or automatic professional courtesy. An inflated sense of entitlement may complicate your relationship with your caregivers.

- Take the time you need to get better. Let your physician manage any administrative pressures from your superiors that may hinder your recovery. Most contracts allow for sick leave so you will not be penalized for absence from work.
- Never self-prescribe medications or order investigations (see the classic article by GE Vaillant: Physician cherish thyself: the hazards of self-prescribing. *JAMA* 1992; 267: 2773–2783).
- If you are HIV-positive yourself, read 'The legal rights and obligations of HIV-infected health care workers' from GLMA (The Gay and Lesbian Medical Association) or contact your provincial or state medical association for current policies.

LEARNING

Effective study seems virtually impossible when you are tired or overworked. Decreased sleep, anxiety, physical discomfort, and high noise and distraction levels have variable effects on the desire to learn, memory, reading capacity, concentration, and task performance. The housestaff member who has a weekend or evening off is unlikely to study because of a need for sleep or social contact; he or she may then feel guilty and inadequate.

Be aware of your preferred learning styles and which one to use in different circumstances. (Most people's learning styles draw on one or two behaviours that they prefer to others.) Knowing this will help you to keep up learning throughout your medical career, and in selecting/ accessing appropriate CME (continuing medical education) options.

BASIC LEARNING STYLES

- using examples from concrete experience (e.g., in-class case studies)
- observing, listening, and reflecting (e.g., after doing rounds)
- working with abstract concepts, relying heavily on logic for analysis and theorizing (e.g., studying texts and debating with colleagues and teachers)
- learning by doing, active experimenting, and practising (e.g., making diagnoses, performing procedures, and working with patients)

Continuing Medical Education: Definitions and Options[16,17]

The AMA and the Accreditation Council for Continuing Medical Education define CME as follows: 'Continuing medical education consists of educational activities that serve to maintain, develop, or increase the knowledge, skills, and professional performance and relationships that a physician uses to provide services for patients, the public, or the profession. The content of CME is that body of knowledge and skills generally recognized and accepted by the profession as within the basic medical sciences, the discipline of clinical medicine, and the provision of health care to the public' (AMA Policy Statement 300.988). The Royal College of Physicians and Surgeons of Canada now requires 'Main Cert' credits for maintenance of certification (see rcpsc.medical.org/english/maintenance). Increasingly, CME will become a mandatory part of maintaining licensing in most jurisdictions.

CONTINUING MEDICAL EDUCATION OPTIONS

Self-directed Methods

- reading journals, texts
- computer programs
- clinical traineeships
- teaching
- publishing
- literature searches
- audio- or videotapes
- self-assessment / needs assessment programs
- research
- self-audit of practice

Group CME Methods

- grand rounds
- conferences
- audits of practice
- structured formal examinations
- journal club
- workshops
- self-assessment programs
- quality assurance programs

Making the Most of Your Learning Potential

1. Identify your own preferred learning style, as described above.
2. During teaching rounds, concentrate on taking away one new fact from each seminar. Learn something new every day.
3. Try to read up on a subject before a lecture to enhance learning.
4. At the beginning of your residency, reading about the cases you are actually treating provides a natural motivation.
5. Carry useful pocket manuals so that concisely organized facts are readily accessible.
6. Subscribe to one or two good peer-reviewed, indexed journals in your field and read the review articles. (See items 17 and 19 in the references at the end of this chapter for an overview of guidelines to selecting, reading, and critiquing the scientific literature.)
7. If a synopsis of your large specialty textbook is available, read it and answer any review questions it contains. Use the large textbook for a more thorough review of a topic.
8. When asked to prepare a grand rounds, pick a practical, non-esoteric topic that you want to learn about. Concentrate on evidence-based clinical articles.
9. Ask to incorporate 'mini rounds' into morning rounds (e.g., a five-minute presentation on a useful topic every morning).
10. Do not be afraid to ask questions during rounds; you are there to learn.
11. Insist on proper supervision by attending staff. Recently the Joint Commission of Accreditation of Healthcare Organization and the ACGME beefed up resident supervision rules, making it mandatory that medical staff be aware of these changes (see www.ama-assn.org/sci-pubs/amnews/pick_01/prsd0709.htm)
12. Carry a notebook to jot down questions and useful facts, pointers, tables, and normal laboratory values.
13. Try to play a teaching role with juniors and medical students; this will force you to review and present data clearly.
14. Identify gaps in your learning. For instance, push for rotations in primary care, 'free' or public health clinics, community and health centres; otherwise your training may be incomplete for practice in a non-hospital setting (i.e., 'the real world').
15. Arrange occasional individual teaching sessions with a mentor or tutor. You may have to request such sessions if your program does not offer them.

16. If your contract allows it, arrange to take time off every year for study, conferences, and exam preparation. Consider using this time to take a specialty review or exam preparation course.

17. Conduct medline searches on topics of interest through your hospital library or by subscribing to a medline vendor service.

TIPS FOR WORLD WIDE WEB/INTERNET MEDICAL LEARNING

- For a wide range of options, check the following entryways:
  www.slackinc.com/matrix
  www.emory.edu/whsci/medweb.html
- Most medical journals can now be found on the Web. Look in journal copies or call your medical library for the addresses.
- Medline, a free Internet searching tool on medical topics, can be found at seven sites, including www.helix.com and www.healthgate.com. PubMed can be found at www.ncbi.nlm.hih.gov/PubMed. Abstracts are free, but there is a fee for ordering full article texts.
- Chatlines/discussion groups are a useful medium for consulting informally with local and international colleagues. Select a subject/group through the following addresses:
  www.altavista.com
  www.reference.com
  www.dejanews.com
- Most university medical schools/research centres have continuing-medical-education sites which offer courses, lectures, problem-based learning, clinical cases, and a chance to exchange ideas. Call the postgraduate medical education office at the university of interest for its Web address.
- As well, most medical associations, specialty groups and societies, and licensing organizations have Web sites which provide information on upcoming meetings, residency issues, and educational seminars. Call for Web site locations.

One of the greatest stresses of residency involves preparing for and then taking the written and oral qualifying exams (the 'Boards') associated with internship, residency, or subspecialty fellowship.

Study/Exam Preparation Tips

- Find out application deadlines for written and oral exams. As the exam draws near, form a study group with three or four friends whose study styles are similar to yours.
- Consider every patient you see to be a potential case presentation for your exam. Discipline yourself to do a thorough history, physical, and case formulation about your patient. Practise presenting the case formally to a teammate from time to time.
- Remember to read about specific cases and actively protect study time throughout your residency.
- Emphasize problem solving rather than memorization, but remember to review rare disease entities and the basic medical sciences of your specialty (i.e., physiology, biochemistry), as you may be asked questions about these in the written and oral exams.
- Try to obtain past fellowship or board written exams and work through them alone or with your study group.
- Find out about board reviews offered by your program or intensive exam workshops offered at other national centres.
- Arrange mock oral exams with senior clinicians in your department at least once a year and request detailed written and verbal feedback.
- Talk to recent candidates about the content/format of their exam.
- To avoid 'study burnout,' reward yourself, for example with outing when you've had a productive session.
- For information on step 3 of the USMLE (United States Medical Licensing Exam), see www.usmle.org.

TEACHING

One of the enduring ironies in postgraduate medical education is that staff physicians teach residents and residents teach medical students, but it seems in most programs that nobody teaches anybody *how* to teach.

Teaching occurs at the bedside, on rounds, in conference rooms, in journal clubs, on grand rounds, and at conferences, but most residents are hard-pressed to describe their own learning style (see above), much less which attributes make an effective teacher. Residents generally emulate 'good teachers' and promise themselves not to be like 'bad teachers.'

Many postgraduate medical offices provide workshops and tutorials on teaching and some staff physicians make a point of teaching about teaching. One useful program offered at centres across Canada and the United States is TIPS (The Teaching Improvement Project System). Here following are practical suggestions for maximizing teaching and learning in a variety of settings.

How to Maximize Bedside Teaching

It is surprising that less than 20 per cent of resident time is actually spent at the bedside, but this time is vital for trainees to learn about patient interviewing, communications skills, and the art of the physical exam.
  Remember to:

- Model respect for the patient's privacy and wishes; keep visits brief.
- Introduce the patient to team members. Express gratitude for their time and assistance in teaching.
- Tell your team members in advance what you want them to observe/ examine regarding the patient, so as not to linger at the bedside unnecessarily.
- Discuss the patient's case in a confidential fashion and setting (i.e., not in the elevator or cafeteria).
- Observe students' or juniors' physical exam and interviewing skills wherever possible and provide immediate, one-on-one feedback.
- Schedule five-minute 'mini-rounds' on a useful topic during every morning round. Seize as many teaching opportunities as you can in the course of the day.
- Work to create a comfortable learning environment where ridicule, criticism, and unhealthy competition are not found. Be open to questions and feedback yourself.

How to Give Verbal Feedback to a Trainee

- Make your expectations known for medical students, interns, and junior residents at the beginning of the rotation and refer to these throughout.
- Always focus your comments on specific performance observations, behaviours, or events rather than making subjective generalizations.
- Find an approximate time and quiet setting for discussion.
- Focus on what needs to be changed. Be succinct and direct and don't provide too much information.

- Frame your comments in an empathic, constructive fashion, emphasizing patient care, teamwork, and common goals for the patient (i.e., to avoid 'put downs,' blaming, or 'ego challenges').
- Make your comments solution-based. Try to have the trainee elicit specific actions/decisions/changes which would result in improved performance.
- Give frequent feedback and follow-up on previous discussions.
- Familiarize yourself with your program's resident evaluation forms so you know what specific elements to look for in a trainee's performance.
- Consult this useful reference: Weinholtz D, Edwards J: *Teaching during Rounds: A Handbook for Attending Physicians and Residents.* Johns Hopkins University Press, Baltimore, 1992.

Maximizing Conference Room Teaching

- Start and finish on time.
- Use audiovisual materials (including x-rays, scans, photographs) wherever possible to illustrate case material.
- Try to keep presentations case-based, rather than lecture-style, as this has been shown to motivate physician learning.
- Use the chalkboard or an overhead projector to graph lab results or draw other graphs.
- If a resident is presenting a case or a topic, let him or her finish with few interruptions, saving questions for the end.
- Summarize key points. Ask Socratic-type questions to stimulate discussion.
- Try to provide handouts, summaries, bibliographies, or review articles at the end of the learning session.

HOW TO GIVE AN EFFECTIVE AUDIOVISUAL PRESENTATION USING SLIDES/OVERHEADS/POWERPOINT[18]

- Do not plan to use more than one slide/overhead per minute or you will overwhelm your audience.
- Number and order your slides carefully. If you can't read your own slide at arm's length, the print is probably too small. Limit the text to one line if possible.

- Use bold print and no more than six lines per slide / six words per line to facilitate reading. Use bullet headings to focus attention.
- Keep graphs and figures simple.
- Consider using dual projectors to contrast images (i.e., before and after treatment), or text versus an image like a CT scan or x-ray.
- Try not to move backwards and forwards with slides. If you need to re-reference a slide have another copy of it placed appropriately in your carousel.
- If using a pointer, be incisive to refer to a specific point; don't 'wander.'
- Arrive in the lecture theatre early to set up and familiarize yourself with the microphone, AV equipment, and light dimmer.
- Turn the lights back on during discussion time.
- Pay attention to timing: begin and end your talk promptly in the allotted time, leaving ample time for questions and feedback.

Other Tips on Presentation/Content

- State the intent of your talk, outline the learning objectives, and make sure your presentation has a beginning, middle, and end.
- Keep content relevant, concise, and interesting without too much detail. Use appropriate humour to engage your audience.
- Practise speaking clearly in a conversational style with good pacing, volume, and pitch. Don't read a script and, wherever possible, try to interact with your audience.
- Dress professionally for the occasion in comfortable, unrestricting clothing.

REFERENCES

1 Colford JM, McPhee SJ: The ravelled sleeve of care: managing the stresses of residency training. *JAMA* 1989; 261: 889–893
2 Leighton K, Livingston M: Fatigue in doctors. *Lancet* 1983; 1: 1280

3 Friedman RC, Bigger JT, Kornfeld DS: The intern and sleep loss. *N Engl J Med* 1971; 285: 201–203

4 Idem: Psychological problems associated with sleep deprivation in interns. *J Med Educ* 1973; 48: 436–441

5 Katz S: Shifting gears: shift work's assault on our biological rhythms. *Med Post* 3 Oct 1989; 11–12, 48. These findings were replicated in a CIR survey reported in March 2001

6 Swift D: Humane schedules for residents, interns helps reduce risk of errors. *Med Post* 26 Sept 1989; 47

7 Patton DV, Landers DR, Agarwal IT: Legal considerations of sleep deprivation among resident physicians. *J Health Law* 2001; 34(3): 377–417

8 Veasey S, Rosen R, Barzansky B, Rosen I, Owens J. Sleep loss and fatigue in residency training: a reappraisal. *JAMA* 2002; 288(9): 1116–1124

9 Blum NJ, Lieu TA: The effects of paging on pediatric resident activities. *American Journal of Diseases of Children* 1992; 146(7): 806–808

10 Cited in *CIR News* Dec 2001

11 Marshall SA, Ruedy J: *On-call Principles and Protocols*. 3rd ed. Saunders, Philadelphia, 2000

12 Borysenko J: *Minding the Body, Mending the Mind*. Bantam, New York, 1988

13 Durso C, George SC: Guns 'n' doctors. *The New Physician* Dec 1994

14 Liss G et al: Violence in the workplace. *J Can Med Assoc* 1994; 151: 1243–1246

15 Steben M: AIDS: preventing HIV infection in health care workers. *J Fam Pract* 1990; 13

16 Audet N: How to manage CME reading time efficiently. *Can J CME* Sept 1995; 83–88

17 Mazmanian, PE: Continuing medical education and the physician as learner: guide to the evidence. *JAMA* 2002; 288(9): 1057–1060

18 Snell L: How to give an effective audiovisual presentation. *Can J CME* Sept 1994; 1–3

19 Guyatt G et al (eds): *Users' Guide to the Medical Literature: Essentials of Evidence-based Clinical Practice*. AMA/JAMA, Chicago, 2002

4. Protecting Your Mental Health

Chapter 3 suggested ways of safeguarding physical health by improving your eating, sleeping, and exercise habits. This chapter discusses two important strategies for protecting your mental health: establishing adequate support systems and maximizing a sense of personal control.

Relationships with family, friends, and colleagues will be discussed in chapter 5 since most residents tend to go to these individuals when experiencing difficulty. Other types of support that you might not have considered are available from the following people, groups, and organizations.

SUPPORT INDIVIDUALS

Family Physician

Surprisingly, many physicians do not have their own physicians, preferring to treat themselves or somehow expecting preferential care from colleagues, often with problematic results. One study of internal-medicine residents in a U.S. school revealed that 37 per cent had no primary care physician and 12 per cent acted as their own doctor![1] Before beginning your training, find a family physician who will treat you as a patient but can adapt to your erratic schedule. He or she can be an invaluable referral source for quick initial assessment and treatment, sick notes, stress management, and support.

Chief Resident

The chief resident should be your advocate, open to feedback about your rotations and a mediator between residents and staff. He or she can initiate you to the conditions and customs in a new hospital or ward setting, arrange coverage when you are absent, ease necessary contacts with superiors, and field your call requests for the night duty roster.

Senior Resident/Fellow

This person can be a source of teaching, support, conflict resolution, and service orientation, and can help you organize your work. Do not hesitate to ask this person questions.

Residency Program Directors

Many residents unfortunately do not get to know their residency program director at either the hospital or the university-program level. This important ally can provide information about rotations, electives, evaluations, exams, training options, and requirements; can handle grievances about rotation abuses, requests for absences, or program changes; and can make recommendations about staff conflicts or learning difficulties. Schedule at least two appointments a year with the program director for feedback and to discuss your progress and career plans.

Hospital Housestaff Association or Resident Representative

This person should address such issues as duties, call frequency, adequacy of supervision, staff relations, leave of absence, benefits, legal protection, and potential political action. Most Canadian teaching hospitals have a representative of the provincial hospital housestaff association in addition to a residency program delegate. Only 15 per cent of U.S. programs are unionized, but your hospital may have residency representatives to the hospital or program administration (see chapter 10 regarding union resources).

Religious Representatives

Scheduling a visit or having lunch with the hospital chaplain, rabbi, or other religious representative can help you to explore existential questions and clarify dilemmas that arise during the dark nights of the soul that many residents experience. Visits from them can also help some patients; ask your patients if they would like a visit arranged.

Hospital Ethics Consultant

Residents may feel ill at ease following certain recommendations of a senior person or experience moral conflicts in treating patients. These circumstances create great stress. Most teaching hospitals and universities have an ethics consultant who can be asked about such cases and invited to give formal or informal seminars.

Hospital Lawyer or Risk Manager

This person can answer questions about consent, confidentiality, incompetence, and termination of treatment, either personally or in requested lectures. Contact with this person is especially important in the United States, where the high risk of malpractice suits lends cogency to arguments for reducing residents' hours and improving working conditions.

Hospital Employee Assistance Programs or the Local Medical Association Hotline or Local Physician Well-being Committee

The people from these services can tell you in confidence how to find help for yourself or your colleagues should someone increasingly resort to drugs or alcohol or to other maladaptive behaviour in response to stress. One example is Ontario's PAIRO Helpline at 1-866-HelpDoc (435-7362).

Other Hospital Professionals

A hospital is a complex organization of professionals and non-professionals working together daily. You can have satisfying, friendly exchanges with any of them. If you can avoid taking a 'physician-in-charge' stance, it is possible to develop relations of collaboration, camaraderie, and even friendship with paging operators, security guards, kitchen and cleaning staff, secretaries, orderlies, and x-ray and laboratory technologists, as well as with nurses, pharmacists, social workers, dietitians, and occupational and physical therapists.

Mentor

Young professionals in any discipline need a mentor (a superior who is guide, tutor, and even friend) to help form their identity. Though some residency programs assign tutors, you may wish or be obliged to find a mentor yourself. In the latter case, ask an inspiring lecturer or attending physician for a meeting or request from the residency program director a list of people with similar clinical and research interests. Mentors are usually but not necessarily older people and may be of the same sex as you. This last characteristic may be an important factor in the process of identification that takes place in such a relationship. Many residents prefer same-sex mentors.

Finding a mentor may be the single most important step you take in obtaining professional support during residency. He or she can encourage you when you feel overwhelmed by your duties, buffer disillusionment, and help you with your career decisions.

A GOOD MENTOR

- is experienced, enthusiastic, sparks your interest, and can skilfully guide your reading and learning;
- provides a role model with respect to manner, professional identity, ethical concerns, and lifestyle, and sees medicine as a vocation, not just a job;
- is patient, non-judgmental, and non-evaluative (is not grading you for your work);
- has artistic, research, and/or clinical interests similar to yours;
- is flexible with time, does not compete with you, and is not threatened by your enthusiasm or intelligence;
- is well connected to resource networks and key workers in your field; and
- will help you choose a subspecialty/fellowship and develop leadership skills.

Psychotherapists

Many residents, particularly those in psychiatry programs, begin a psychotherapeutic exploration during residency, often as a result of crisis (substance abuse, depression, or decreasing performance) and sometimes because they believe such work will make them happier people and better physicians. Your family physician, residency program director, hospital or provincial or state physician well-being committee, physician hotline, or you yourself, privately, can usually arrange a referral. Some residency programs include counselling networks.

Select a therapist carefully; as one psychiatrist observed, 'You don't get to pick your parents, so you'd better be careful finding a therapist.' Interview prospective therapists about philosophy and length of treatment, an active versus a silent approach, availability of a professional rate, and flexibility of hours, all the while assessing personal fit or compatibility ('Is this someone I can talk to?'). Decide whether you want support or a perceptive examination of conflicts, and whether you want short-term work or to keep the therapy open-ended. Make a contract with the therapist that sets goals, expectations, and basic ground rules (rates, attendance, holidays, cancellations, etc.).

The logistics of attending therapy sessions during residency are complex but not impossible. If your residency program director has provided the referral, he or she may help you to be seen quickly and can be quoted during rotations as supporting therapy work. The referral source and therapist will keep your work confidential, but you will still have to explain absences to your senior or chief resident. Explain only as much as you want, but at the least that your work should not suffer from regular one- to two-hour absences each week. Having a therapist in the same hospital or nearby is an obvious advantage. Remember to keep any receipts for income tax purposes and to discuss with your therapist whether treatment will restrict medical/disability insurance access later on.

SUPPORT GROUPS[2]

Resident Support Groups (General)

Some very worthwhile friendships form during internship and residency because of the intensity of the shared experience, the similar goals, and the countless hours residents spend together. Many residents unfortunately miss the opportunity of giving and receiving informal peer support because they are competitive or believe they have to appear all-knowing and omnipotent. They are reluctant to discuss anxiety, sickness, self-doubt, or feelings of failure and loss. Allow yourself to let off steam, because it will help open exchange and normalize the many feelings that get stirred up in all residents during training. Ask for help when you need it, cover for each other, do favours, talk through intense shared experiences together (like the death of a patient). Build in play time. All these activities are rewarding and protective. When you are a senior, look out for those under you, recognize their anxiety, and ask them to talk about such key experiences as the first night of call. Be a role model by showing that residents should talk about such things. Always set up an orientation for new interns or new residents on your service.

The literature on resident stress and impairment has established the usefulness of a variety of formal group experience for residents.[3] Women's groups, spouses' groups, couples' groups, trainee-staff retreats, first-year orientation weeks or months, medical society memberships, process or

Balint-type groups, and peer/process support groups have all been used with success in teaching centres across North America. They may be optional or an established part of the program, time-limited or open, led by a behavioural scientist or self-run, and held weekly, monthly, or semi-annually. Interns in particular benefit from such groups because they help to manage the stress of the first postgraduate year.

U.S. Resident Support Structure – What's Ideal?

The ACGME now requires that support services be available to all residents. Dr Robert Levey in his recent literature review in *Academic Medicine*[4] highlights the stressors cited previously in chapter 1, but also mentions the dilemmas faced by IMGs, residents who are matched to programs they don't want, pregnant and minority residents, and those with learning difficulties. He describes the following ingredients of an ideal assistance service:

- confidentiality
- support from program staff
- short-term counselling for trainees and their family members
- an objective third-party referral service
- ongoing follow-up for severely stressed residents
- social activities/retreats
- support groups for residents and family members
- stress seminars
- child care / financial resources

The various residency program syllabuses and information networks now list and describe the support programs available at every hospital or university setting. See chapter 10 ('Resources') for information on FREIDA (The Fellowship and Residency Electronic Interactive Database). All of this information should figure highly in the choice of a program.

Housestaff Associations

Political support and influence are necessary to change the many stressful conditions now prevalent in the residency experience. All Canadian residents are employed by provincial agencies and represented by provincial housestaff associations, which provide uniform contracts. The Canadian Association of Interns and Residents (CAIR) has been serving as the umbrella organization for provincial housestaff associations (excluding the Fédération des Médecins résidents du Québec [FMRQ]) since 1970.

The CAIR's executive committee consists of provincially elected members who meet three times a year in different Canadian cities and sit on several of the major medical bodies, including the Canadian Medical Association (CMA), the Canadian Medical Protective Association (CMPA), the Royal College of Physicians and Surgeons of Canada (RCPSC), and various government committees (e.g., national manpower). The CAIR publishes the *Canadian Housestaff* newsletter and other communications, which residents can request. The CAIR has also been active in sharing its expertise with its U.S. counterparts.

The situation in the United States is unfortunately entirely different. Residents are generally hired and paid by their specific hospital centre, and only 25 per cent have housestaff unions with collective agreements. The CIR (the Committee of Interns and Residents [1-800-247–8877; www.cirseiu.org]) is the oldest, largest housestaff union in the United States, with chapters across the country, and has an affiliation with SEIU (the Service Employees' International Union), which is the single largest American union of health employees. The CIR's services include consultation and advice on contract negotiations, union formation, and policies on call duties, licensing, funding, debt repayment, and other housestaff issues (i.e., quality of training and quality of life for patients and residents). The CIR publishes a newspaper, *CIR News*,[5] which monitors these concerns and carries information packets on affirmative action, international medical graduate rights, legislative issues, public-sector health care, contract negotiation, parenting issues, setting up a housestaff organization, limiting hours, and issues like residency and AIDS.

Other examples of more local unions can be found at the University of Michigan and the University of Colorado, as well as specific county hospitals (like Cook County Hospital in Chicago). Other schools and hospitals have housestaff associations which organize collectively on behalf of residents, but don't bargain and are not recognized under the National Labor Relations Act, as unions are.

Other residents in the United States are not protected in any systematic way from local abuses in working conditions, especially in the southern states. Many residents have no board representation at the administrative level in the hospitals where they work. Challenges to contract violation must be fought individually. As well, many states and hospital corporations choose to see residents as students rather than employees, thereby blocking the possibility for union formation and recognition. Nonetheless, many residents are ambivalent about what unionization means within a profession like medicine and what impact it has on the doctor–patient relationship.

The American Medical Association plays a significant role in the lives of residents in the United States. Its Resident and Fellow Section (RFS), with over 35,000 members, is the largest organization of residents in the United States and contributes directly to the AMA policy-making process. Its journal (*JAMA*) publishes a regular column called 'On Call' (email, oncall@ama-assn.org) which highlights key developments affecting young physicians in terms of legislation, debt repayment, practice formation, and training. In 1997, the AMA created its own union called Physicians for Responsible Negotiation (PRN), whose policies contained a no-strike clause. The AMA also offers expert speakers to help residents explore their representational options (for information call 312-464-4750 or consult the AMA website, www.ama-assn.org).

Other organizations of interest to interns and residents in the United States include:

- AMSA (the American Medical Student Association), which describes itself as 'the largest and oldest independent association representing physicians-in-training, including pre-medical students, medical students, interns and residents. Founded in 1950 to provide an opportunity for medical students to participate in organized medicine, AMSA began as the Student American Medical Association under the auspices of the American Medical Association (AMA). In 1967, AMSA formally ended its affiliation with the AMA and has since remained an independent organization. Governed by a student Board of Trustees, much of the association's energy today is focused on reforming the medical education system, improving work conditions and developing physician leadership for the 21st century. AMSA has nearly 30,000 members in 168 chapters.' Its headquarters is located at 1890 Preston White Drive, Reston, Virginia.[6]
- The ACGME (Accreditation Council for Graduate Medical Education) is the only accrediting body for the more than 6,000 residency training programs in the United States. Representatives from the AMA, the American Board of Medical Specialties, the American Hospital Association, and the Association of American Medical Colleges, along with resident representatives and representatives from the public sector and the federal government, make up this body. The ACGME insists that every residency program have a grievance policy overseen by the

hospital graduate medical education committee. It also investigates complaints about programs.

- The AAMC (Association of American Medical Colleges) has an Organization of Resident Representatives who discuss issues pertinent to resident well-being.

Residents considering their options with respect to forming unions, housestaff associations, or other resident for a can consult the agencies listed above. Increasingly these organizations are collaborating and 'cross-pollenating' to improve conditions for residents nation-wide.

Setting Up Your Own Support Group

- Establish resident interest in attending a group and determine feasible frequency. Offer food!
- Approach the program director for expertise, suggestions, and funding if a mental health professional is to lead the group. The director's support is necessary, particularly if residents are to be freed from their duties to attend.
- Decide whether the group is to be self-led or led by a non-evaluating faculty member or mental health professional. It is a good idea to have a leader, especially at the beginning, to help build trust.
- Plan logistics carefully. Aim for weekly or biweekly meetings lasting forty-five to sixty minutes, possibly over lunch, and attended by seven to ten people. Arrange coverage for those attending and provide food. Consider holding a resident retreat away from the hospital once or twice a year.
- Prepare and publicize a list of resources for emergency care should members need outside help.
- Remember your goals: the group provides support, not psychotherapy. It will help members to air their feelings ('gripe sessions'), normalize stresses, and solve problems. Topics can be chosen in advance, or pressing concerns can guide the format of each meeting. The amount of self-relevation will vary, but the focus should be on shared problem solving regarding residency stresses and on physician–patient and physician–staff relations. Members should speak for themselves, not for each other.
- Prepare a list of ten to twelve difficult situations/scenarios that residents are likely to face in training (i.e., verbal abuse, arranging organ donation, facing a clinical error).
- A good group leader will encourage but not teach or guide content,

and will defuse conflict and comment on process only if it impedes members' giving mutual support. (The leader may be more active, interpreting underlying conflicts, if the group is an experiential or process one.)

- Speakers can be invited, and films shown. Topics for discussion can include burnout, fatigue, the 'difficult patient,' resident competence versus fear of error and failure, the dying patient, bearing bad news, handling staff conflict, ethical dilemmas, the impaired resident, stress-management techniques, career and financial planning, balancing family life, and a review of local, provincial or state, and national resources. See the list at the end of chapter 5 for films, videos, and literature that will prompt discussion on physician identity.
- An online support/chat group can be found at www.wardrounds.com/ wardboards.php. Other websites to share with colleagues include the Internship and Residency Information Site (IRIS), www.i-r-i-s.com/ iris.html; www.MedWebPlus (subject: Internship and Residency); www.studentdoctor.net; and www.pairo.org/wellbeing/resources.html.

MAXIMIZING A PERSONAL SENSE OF CONTROL[6]

Many aspects of residency are beyond your immediate control – for example, hours worked, on-call schedules, rotation content, and exam requirements – but it is surprising to what degree you can be in control of your training if you are motivated and plan carefully. In a sense, doing so provides a form of self-support.

Tips for Keeping Control

- Try to plan your rotation schedule, aiming to alternate between difficult and easy, in- and outpatient rotations. Submit your request to your residency director well in advance.
- Find out the names and rotation schedules of good senior residents and attending physicians and try to arrange to work on their services.
- Obtain a list of hospital statutory holidays and request some long weekends off well in advance.
- Plan and schedule holiday time well in advance; it provides an important respite and should be used strategically.
- Choose hospital assignments that require less call or home call. If possible, live close to the hospital, thereby saving travel time and increasing sleep time.
- Keep track of all night calls, particularly weekend or statutory holiday

calls, so that you can request compensation for extras if appropriate. Inform your residency director or housestaff representative of contractual abuses.

- Remember the seasonal nature of rotations and plan accordingly (e.g., the pediatric outpatient department is flat in the summer, and surgery is slow at Christmas).
- Maximize elective time by arranging interesting locations and subject matter. Do not be afraid to request something or somewhere original, and document all arrangements by letter.
- Pamper yourself when you are stressed; for example, take a taxi, order out, hire a cleaner, buy yourself flowers, call long distance to a friend.
- Control your learning. Ask questions and request increased teaching, supervision, or lectures. Ask for one-on-one instruction if you need it.
- Be aware of all the benefits available to you through the hospital and university: library and sports facilities, legal and financial advisers, leaves of absence. Use allotted conference times to learn, explore new locations, and make valuable contacts. Professional, specialty, or society meetings are often inspiring.
- Sometimes crossing each day off on a calendar is a satisfying symbol of getting through. Buy a one-year calendar to record holidays and rotations. Note paydays, special occasions, and deadlines (e.g., references for jobs and exam applications).
- Plan your time every day, listing priorities and 'scut' work and eliminating unnecessary tasks. Order consultations, tests, and support staff services (e.g., electrocardiograms and intravenous drips) early in the day when they are available. Save yourself travel time by developing a system for doing all work (e.g., x-rays) floor by floor or department by department. Make lists when you feel you are losing control, and note pros and cons and options. Consider keeping a journal, or jot down milestones or key events (like 'first delivery,' 'first solo rescuscitation') on your calendar for a personal record of your journey through residency.
- Make a list with your colleagues of 'time drainers' on your service (disorganized sign-outs, lack of access to computers, delays contacting insurance companies), and problem solve together to find and prioritize solutions.
- Remember that you are entitled to sick days, which can be taken when you are feeling particularly under stress. Do not be irresponsible to resident colleagues, but consider taking a 'mental health day,' which will allow you to return rested and more effective.

- Some programs tolerate leaves of absence lasting from twenty days to three months without penalty at the discretion of the residency program director. Keep this option in mind if things get out of hand, and discuss it with the director.
- Take rotation evaluations seriously and do not sign one that you disagree with. Request clarification or rewording rather than waiting for surprises; request regular feedback if you are not getting it during rotations.
- Periodically ask for access to your personnel file to verify its content/ accuracy.
- Obtain a copy of your hospital or union contract and read it carefully. Know what is expected of you and what protection you can expect.
- Remember to keep your options open. Learn the requirements for a general licence so that you can take outside work. Find out the varying provincial and state requirements for internship and residency and keep copies of all correspondence should these requirements change.
- If you are disappointed or overwhelmed, you can attempt to change programs or hospital bases as other positions become vacant (check the specialty journals), sometimes even in mid-year.
- Get political. Consider running for a position in your hospital/CAIR/ provincial (state) housestaff association or union; or as chief resident, faculty representative; regional representative to your specialty association; regional AMA resident physician representative in the United States; or representative to the university or to the university's committee on residency training.
- Find out about physician well-being groups in your area. Talk to the hospital program director about setting up resident-staff feedback (or 'gripe sessions'), a resident support group, or a resident peer review system in which residents participate in evaluating each other's progress and in selecting new candidates of the residency program. If you are a U.S. trainee and there is no union at your hospital, talk about starting one.
- List your goals: professional, personal, romantic, family, financial, spiritual, physical, and so on. Decide to what degree you have attained some of them and what now prevents you from attaining others. Pay attention to your creative side and to how music, literature, and film relax you and enrich your interactions with and understanding of patients. (A medical humanities bibliography [medical history and literature] is provided at the end of this chapter.)

- Consider keeping a journalor writing narrative about your ward experiences as ways to promote self-reflection.
- Know and develop your personal coping skills. Chatting with others, humour, naps, exercise, and leisure time help reduce stress. Determine which activities are most effective for you and build them into your schedule, even if it means sometimes saying 'no' at home and at work.
- Reframe a tendency towards self-criticism by identifying one satisfying event or exchange every day. Remember: you know more today than you did yesterday. Try to live day to day, because you cannot delay gratification indefinitely.
- Get involved in evaluating the care provided in your hospital/department by offering to sit on a quality assessment/assurance board.
- Join a local, national, or Internet health reform group.
- Check your personnel file regularly to make sure it's accurate, balanced and up to date.
- Complete all professor and rotation evaluations. This is not a hopeless gesture but an important source of feedback for program change. If your program doesn't have them, develop the forms yourself. Figure 4.1 is a sample form which can be adapted for use in your program setting.

Figure 4.1 Faculty of Medicine Evaluation of Service by Housestaff

NAME: **LEVEL OF TRAINING:**
SERVICE: **HOSPITAL:**
DATE:

---

1. YOUR WORK LOAD AND CLINICAL RESPONSIBILITY ON SERVICE

a) Number of (on average)	Far Too Few	Too Few	Right	Too Many	Far Too Many
Inpatients					
Clinics					
Consultations					
Emergency Calls					

b) Clinical Responsibility

c) Night Call	1. Nights/month
	2. Average number of hours of sleep you got

2. YOUR LEARNING EXPERIENCE ON SERVICE

	Needs a Lot of Improvement	Needs Improvement	Good But Could Be Improved	Very Good But Could Be Improved in Some Areas (See Comments)	Excellent
a) Quality of Teaching:					
At Bedside					
On Ward					
In Emergency					
At Subspecialty Rounds					
Evaluation Procedures					
Opportunity to Attend Teaching Sessions					

Comments:

b) Amount of:					
Didactic					
Informal Teaching					
Bedside Teaching					

3. MORALE ON SERVICE

	Needs a Lot of Improvement	Needs Improvement	Good But Could Be Improved	Very Good but Could Be Improved in Some Areas (See Comments)	Excellent
Interaction with:					
Attending Staff					
Nursing Staff					
Other Housestaff					

Comments:

4. TEACHER
% of Rotation Application

	Needs a Lot of Improvement	Needs Improvement	Good But Could Be Improved	Very Good But Could Be Improved in Some Areas (See Comments)	Excellent
Enthusiasm/ Stimulation of Interest					
Clarity and Organization of Teaching					
Availability/ Supervision					
Bedside Teaching					
Ward Rounds					
Seminars (Small Group)					
Procedures					
Interpersonal Skills with Housestaff					
Interpersonal Skills with Patients					

Comments:

5. ON THIS ROTATION YOU WERE TAUGHT

	Needs a Lot of Improvement	Needs Improvement	Good But Could Be Improved	Very Good But Could Be Improved in Some Areas (See Comments)	Excellent
Research Methodology					
About Research					
Critical Appraisal					
Ethics					

Comments:

6. Were education resources (books, reprints, etc.) available and appropriate for this rotation? Please suggest useful additions to the library.

7. Do you think your experience provided you with the education which you desired and which will be relevant to your anticipated clinical practice? Please suggest areas of strength and areas which need improvement in the program.

8. OVERALL EVALUATION OF THS ROTATION

Needs a Lot of Improvement	Needs Improvement	Good But Could Be Improved	Very Good But Could Be Improved in Some Areas (See Comments)	Excellent

Comments:

9. OTHER COMMENTS

Source: Susan L. Moffatt, MD, FRCPC. Reprinted with permission.

REFERENCES

1 Rosen IM, Christie JD, Bellini LM, Asch DA. Health and health care among housestaff in four U.S. internal medicine residency programs. *J Gen Intern Med* 2000; 15(2): 116–121

2 Siegel B, Donnelly JC: Enriching personal and professional development: the experience of a support group for interns. *J Med Educ* 1978; 53: 908–914

3 Tokarz JP, Bremer W, Peter K: *Beyond Survival: A Book Prepared by and for Resident Physicians to Meet the Challenge of the Impaired Physician and to Promote Well-being through Medical Education*, Am Med Assoc, Chicago, 1979

4 Levey RE: Sources of stress for residents and recommendations for programs to assist them. *Academic Medicine* 2001; 76(2): 142–150

5 Committee on Interns and Residents: *News* Mar 1990; 19: 4–5

6 Howell JB, Schroeder DP (eds): *Physician Stress. A Handbook for Coping.* Univ Park Pr, Baltimore, 1984

ADDITIONAL READING

Brady, DW: What's important to you? The use of narratives to promote self-reflection and to understand the experiences of medical residents. *Ann Int Med* 2002; 137(3): 220–223

Kahn N Jr, Schaeffer H: A process group approach to stress reduction and personal growth in a family practice residency program. *J Fam Pract* 1981; 12: 1043–1047

Matthews DA, Classen DC, Willms JL: A program to help interns cope with stresses in an internal medicine residency. *J Med Educ* 1988; 63: 539–547

Rabow MW: Doctoring to heal: fostering well-being among physicians through personal reflection. *West J Med* 2001; 174(1): 66–69

Remen, RN: Recapturing the soul of medicine: physicians need to reclaim meaning in their working lives. *West J Med* 2001; 174(1): 4–5

Scott CD, Hawk J (eds): *Heal Thyself. The Health of Health Care Professionals.* Brunner/Mazel, New York, 1986

Sotile WM, Sotile, MD: *The Resilient Physician: Effective Emotional Management for Doctors and Their Medical Organizations.* AMA Press, Chicago, 2002 (see also www.TheResilientPhysician.ca)

Medical History and Literature

Ackerknecht E: *A Short History of Medicine*, rev ed., Johns Hopkins Univ Pr, Baltimore, 1982

Boussel P: *Histoire de médecine et la chirurgie de la grande peste à nos jours.* Porte verte, Paris, 1979

Brody H: *Stories of Sickness.* Yale Univ Pr, New Haven, 1987

Coles R: *The Call of Stories.* Houghton Mifflin, Boston, 1989

Greenhalgh T, Hurwitz B (eds): *Narrative Based Medicine: Dialogue and Discourse in Clinical Practice.* BMS Books, London, 1998

Inglis B: *A History of Medicine.* Weidenfeld and Nicolson, London, 1965

King LS: *Medical Thinking: A Historical Preface.* Princeton Univ Pr, Princeton, 1982

Kleiman A: *The Illness Narratives: Suffering, Healing and the Human Condition.* Basic Books, New York, 1988

Lyons AS: *Medicine: An Illustrated History.* Abrams, New York, 1978

Shryock R: *The Development of Modern Medicine: An Interpretation of the Social and Scientific Factors Involved.* Univ Wisconsin Pr, Madison, 1974

Trautman J, Pollard C: *Literature and Medicine: An Annotated Bibliography*, 2nd ed. Univ of Pittsburgh Pr, Pittsburgh, 1982

Other Residency Resources on the Web

American Medical Association: www.ama-assn.org/ama/pub/category/5030.html

American Medical Student Association: www.amsa.org/resource/resdir/reshome.cfm

American Osteopathic Association: www.aoa-net.org/Students/students.htm
DocInTraining.com: www.docintraining.com
FindAResident: services.aamc.org/findaresident
National Resident Matching Program: www.nrmp.org
Scutwork.com: www.scutwork.com

5. Protecting Personal and Professional Relationships

COUPLE LIFE

The stresses of training that tax residents will also affect their couple life. Residents' lack of time, exhaustion, absence, and unavailability often produce conflict at home. Because most residents' partners also work outside the home,[1] scheduling of quality time and household duties is complex. Historically, wives of physicians score high on interpersonal sensitivity, depression, and hostility scales.[2] Husbands of physicians may feel threatened by their wives' success, level of responsibility, or income and decision-making power. In his book *Doctors' Marriages: A Look at the Problems and Their Solutions*,[3] Myers points out that the key stressors for the married resident often depend on the developmental level of the couple (e.g., newly married versus settled, childless versus with children).

Large educational debts, the increasingly uncertain future of some specialties, and moonlighting for extra cash at the expense of free time also make money a significant issue for couples.

Moving to another city adds pressures to relationships. Residents find that getting started in their training program can give a stimulating and structured focus to relocating. Their partners, however, may feel ambivalent about the move and burdened by the logistics. They can feel isolated, and lonely for friends and family in the new city. Social life gradually diminishes because there is little time to see other couples or family members. The common-law, gay, other-race, or recently immigrated partner of a resident may feel particularly stigmatized in a conservative medical social milieu or general community. Some couples are geographically separated by the Match and try to maintain long-distance relationships, which involve their own stressors.[4]

The resident's personality may change so much during training (e.g., with a tendency towards irritability, hypersensitivity, or overconfidence) that the partner may feel abandoned. Residents concerned about their career choice or competence may become more preoccupied and withdrawn, and may shut out their partners because of feelings of shame and failed responsibility. The high levels of resident exhaustion can cause changes in the quality of a couple's sex life, which the partner may perceive as rejection. Partners may also believe that their concerns are dwarfed by those of physicians who are diligently saving lives and who have grown accustomed to adopting a direct and authoritative stance. Many residents even develop a psychiatric illness (see chapter 1), which may precipitate or aggravate conflict in the relationship.

Decisions that are usually shared, such as the timing of having children and settling versus moving, become more complicated for both partners, particularly for women physicians, who experience 'role strain' (the wish to be 'super' physicians, mothers, wives, and daughters). Household tasks and raising children often constitute the most frequent sources of resident couple conflict. Unfortunately, medical colleagues may not acknowledge the value of male residents' trying to reduce the risks of conflict by participating in these tasks.

AVOIDING TROUBLE IN COUPLE LIFE[5]

- Remember that your partner is not medically trained and may need frequent explanations about expectations, scientific terms, causes of stress, procedures, and duties; however, avoid constant shop talk.
- Write out a schedule of shifts and rotations with probable hours so your partner knows what to expect. Make a list of household tasks with your partner and discuss how to share them, taking into account each other's workloads.
- Plan time alone together in advance rather than hoping it will happen. Go out on a 'date' at least once a week!
- Leave the job at the hospital. Avoid constant calls to the hospital or worrying about things you might have forgotten.
- Acknowledge when you are tired, angry, or sad, and state the source of the feeling (the job, home, or elsewhere).
- Set aside a regular time to talk about your priorities and long-term goals as a couple, emphasizing things to look forward to.

- Call home at least once a shift.
- Do things to increase closeness: have dinner together at the hospital on a call night, telephone each other, leave notes, arrange surprises, buy gifts, make playful gestures.
- Develop shared hobbies and activities: sports, gardening, home improvement, family visits, and so forth.
- Maximize support from family, friends, social events, and residency resources.

SIGNS OF TROUBLE IN COUPLE LIFE[3]

- increased quarrelling, particularly over 'picky' issues
- decreased relating (talking, sex, leisure, play, or vacation time)
- avoidant behaviours
- sexual infidelity
- fear of 'nothing left in common'
- symptoms of anxiety, depression, or substance abuse in either or both partners
- increased unresolved anger or anger exhibited passively or violently

Dealing with Conflict[3]

- Label problems in a non-accusatory way.
- Use 'we' rather than 'you' in discussions.
- Separate internal (couple) issues from external ones (e.g., residency time pressures).
- Listen openly and avoid a defensive stance or attitude.
- Acknowledge that problems may be situational or temporary, but do not pretend they will simply disappear.
- Refer your partner to the International Medical Spouse Network, an online support/discussion group – www.geocities.com/medicalspouse/survey1.html.
- Try to develop mutual support and support from family, friends, and other couples.
- Protect or add time for talking, play, sex, and vacations.

• Investigate options such as residency support groups, marriage retreats, and counselling through your religious community, resident
services, or the hospital department of psychiatry or psychology.

Should You Medically Treat a Friend or Family Member?[6]

In order to avoid potential complications and the boundary blurring
inherent in caring for family and friends, here are key questions to ask
yourself before doing so.

1. Does my relative's presenting problem fall into my area of expertise?
   Am I trained/equipped to deal with the problem?
2. Am I equipped to deal with a relative's personal or sexual history in
   an objective way? Could I deliver bad news or a poor prognosis
   honestly if required?
3. Am I objective enough not to defensively overtreat, or not to use
   denial regarding the severity of the problem and undertreat?
4. If I help a particular family member medically, what effect will this
   have on family conflicts, patterns, or dynamics?
5. Will my friend or family member do as I suggest (comply with treatment) or take advice less seriously because of the personal connection?
6. Will I, through anxiety or a sense of entitlement, interfere with care
   once my friend or family member is referred on to a colleague?
7. Am I willing to be held accountable ethically and medicolegally if my
   care is judged substandard, incomplete, or inadequate?

Generally, with the exception of emergencies, it is preferrable to refer a
family member to a colleague. If you decide to provide care, raise the
above issues with the individual in order to establish a working, doctor–
patient relationship, then proceed with caution.

PARENTING

This section is addressed principally to women residents; however, their
partners and other supportive colleagues who share the responsibilities
of parenting should learn to appreciate the importance of the issues and
the suggestions they present. Happily, male residents are increasingly
making use of paternity leave as well.

• During parental leave, keep up to date by reading journals in your
specialty and consider the rewards of returning to work you do well;
do not view your return to residency as the enemy.

- Investigate child-care options (day care, in-home babysitting, or live-in help).
- Given irregular work schedules and the frequency of childhood illnesses, remember the need for back-up; day-care centres tend to have fixed drop-off and pick-up times. When hiring at-home help, interview applicants with your partner and check all references. Look for someone with a flexible attitude towards duties (including cooking and light housekeeping), availability, and hours; procedures on rotations and rounds will make the timing of your arrival home unpredictable. Before you finish your maternity leave, arrange to observe how candidates interact with your child. Do not scrimp or rush when hiring a caregiver with whom your child will form a significant bond. You must be satisfied that the relationship will be a good one.
- Remember that a portion of child-care costs is tax creditable; keep receipts.
- Because residency hours tend to be inflexible, flexibility at home is important. Discuss and agree with your partner on how to share the parenting responsibilities, and try to arrange elective rotations with flexible hours for your return after maternity leave.
- Ask your attending physician to finish rounds at a reasonable hour and arrange coverage with another resident for emergencies.
- For family emergencies, recruit other support for your role as a parent among friends, neighbours, family, and in-laws by asking them to help and to visit your child regularly.
- Ask colleagues with children for other strategies.
- Carry a beeper so that your caregiver can reach you in emergencies (you will feel more comfortable knowing that you are available) and call home every day to say 'hi' to older children.
- Establish regular rituals with your children to ensure quality time with them; when you come home tired at the end of the day, for example, try a five-minute cuddle session. Set a time that follows your own rest period for playing or reading stories.
- Make your 'off-call' time inviolate for your family; plan holiday time in advance, even if you stay home, so that the whole family has something to look forward to.
- Try to do your reading at work, because it will be next to impossible at home.
- Avoid a tendency to reproach yourself for not being the ideal parent-physician. You and your family *will* survive the rigours of residency!

Other Parenting Resources

The following resources will assist you in exploring options and decision making as a working parent:

Day Care: Finding the Best Child Care for Your Family, a booklet published by the American Academy of Pediatrics. To order, write: AAP/Dept. C/IH, 141 NW Point Blvd, Elk Grove, IL 60007.

Medicine and Parenting, a booklet published by the Association of American Medical Colleges.

Building a Stronger Women's Program, which includes a chapter on flexibility related to parenting. To order this and the previous resource, write: AAMC Publication Sales, Suite 200, One Dupont Circle NW, Washington, DC 20036.

Questions about discrimination, parental leave, and related issues may be directed to the Gender Equity Hotline, a referral service offered by the American Medical Women's Association. Call (703) 838-0500.

THE SINGLE RESIDENT

Residents who are single and live alone may be at increased emotional risk because of lack of support mechanisms; they may become increasingly isolated socially because they have little time or energy to meet new people or to date. They may also be reluctant to acknowledge feelings of loneliness to themselves or others because such feelings are not part of their self-concept as competent professionals. Most of their initial social contacts come from the hospital, because they are often in a new city, and their schedule tends to keep them from exploring. For some residents, this is not a happy prospect.

COPING MECHANISMS FOR SINGLE RESIDENTS

- Remember your need for support from family and friends throughout residency, and avoid the tendency to withdraw socially when fatigued or to deny feelings of loneliness.
- Attend hospital social events, especially at the beginning of residency. You have to start socializing sometime, and you will meet other, non-hospital-affiliated people at these occasions.
- Make it a rule not to talk shop with medical friends at social

---

occasions. Cultivate non-medical friends through sports, hobbies, or religious groups.

- If you live alone, buy an answering machine so that you do not miss invitations.
- Consider renting or requesting a beeper for the year to give yourself more flexibility to leave the hospital, take a break, or be more available to friends and family.
- Consider joining a health club, a religious group, your building's tenants' association, or special-interest or political groups, realizing, however, that you may have to miss some meetings.
- Make yourself go out socially, even if you're tired.
- Consider living with a compatible medical or non-medical roommate. Establish clear rules about quiet time (post-call), sharing chores, and so on.
- Schedule vacations with friends well in advance so that you have something to look forward to.
- Request your call nights well in advance so that you can plan your social life (e.g., special concerts and long weekends away).
- Maintain links with family members, even if they live in another city, through visits, frequent telephone calls, and e-mail.

Should You Date a Patient?[7]

In today's medicolegal environment, socializing with patients may be ill advised because of accusations of boundary violations.

Here are some suggested guidelines regarding romantic or sexual involvement with a patient. Check with your local medical/professional association or licensing body for up-to-date local recommendations.

- Sexual relationships between patients in active (current) treatment and doctors must be avoided.
- A period of time (usually one year) should lapse between the date of the last medical follow-up with the patient and the onset of the romantic or sexual contact.
- Where treatment involved psychoanalysis, psychotherapy, or extensive counselling, sexual or romantic involvement with the patient

should be avoided (and is prohibited by many professional associations).

- Special caution should be exercised before a physician starts dating a former patient if the professional context with the patient resulted in the patient's emotional dependency on the doctor or created any other vulnerability which may have impaired the patient's judgment or ability to make free decisions.
- Pay attention to how long you've known the patient, what care you've provided, and other relevant circumstances before dating. If in doubt, consult an impartial colleague or psychotherapist.

OTHER RESIDENTS

Impaired housestaff team relations usually go undetected by staff supervisors and are usually not addressed by residents themselves.[8] The results are increased anxiety for team members and, ultimately, compromised patient care. The varieties of resident personalities and associated interactive styles significantly affect the development of housestaff teams, as does the tendency of residents to hide worries from each other in an attempt to appear competent. Attending physicians may be absent most of the time, and senior or chief residents may be unaccustomed to a leadership and teaching role or more interested in exploiting their new position in the hospital hierarchy to reduce their own workload. Conflict is not defused in such circumstances.

SIGNS OF TROUBLE AMONG RESIDENTS[8]

- increased sarcasm
- increased petty disagreements over esoteric points
- formation of factions and scapegoating
- increased sick leave, lateness, and longer rounds
- decreased morale and increased anger, depression, and fatigue in team members
- decreased attendance and helpfulness in teaching and coverage
- power struggles (e.g., changing others' orders)
- unfinished work (a risk to patients)

DEALING WITH TEAM TROUBLES

• Define the problem (e.g., external stress or interpersonal tension).
• Arrange an initial team meeting to let off steam ('gripe sessions').
• Keep the discussion 'team-' or 'we-' oriented rather than accusing people. Talk about behaviours, not personalities.
• If the initial meeting is unsuccessful, recruit the attending physician, senior resident, or a hospital mediator to intervene.

PREVENTING CONFLICT

• Encourage team support by acknowledging shared moments of stress and anxiety.
• Schedule prophylactic mid-rotation 'gripe sessions' for stressful rotations (e.g., in intensive care or surgery).
• Introduce appropriate humour to rounds.
• Consider arranging occasional dinner or social meetings outside the hospital.

Often conflict between residents on different teams/services occurs because of unclear requests or expectations, 'turf wars,' or patient 'dumping,' when one team wants to transfer care. Here are some suggestions for effective consulting/liaison.

AVOIDING TURF WARS: TEN COMMANDMENTS FOR EFFECTIVE CONSULTATION[9]

1. Determine the consultation question – call the consultee when necessary.
2. Establish urgency – emergent, urgent, or routine.
3. Look for yourself – examine the patient, review old data, and

collect new information. Summarize lab/key test data for
yourself.
4. Be as brief as appropriate – there is no need to repeat in full
    detail the data already recorded in the chart. Provide a pri-
    mary and differential diagnosis.
5. Be specific, brief, and goal-oriented regarding treatment
    recommendations.
6. Provide a prognonsis and contingency plans – anticipate
    potential problems. Offer a 'decision tree' for problem
    solving.
7. Honour thy turf – don't take over the patient's care, unless
    requested to do so.
8. Teach with tact – give references and communicate impor-
    tant information courteously and personally.
9. Provide direct personal contact – especially if recommenda-
    tions are crucial or potentially controversial.
10. Follow up – provide suggestions for follow-up in the hospi-
    tal and make suggestions for arranging outpatient care.

THE IMPAIRED COLLEAGUE

How to deal with a colleague who is impaired poses a serious medical
and ethical dilemma for physicians who feel torn between protecting a
friend or colleague and protecting the patients that person serves. First,
how do you distinguish between stress and impairment? Signs of impairment or burnout that exceed the intermittent symptoms of fatigue
include:

• unexplained lateness and absence
• carelessness, indifference, apathy, and increased mistakes in patient
  care
• visible drug or alcohol abuse; pervasive clinical symptoms of anxiety,
  depression, psychosis (paranoia), mania, impaired memory, talk of
  suicide, and hopelessness
• increased preoccupation with marital or professional conflicts
• decreased efficiency (unfinished work, sometimes despite longer hours)
• increased angry outbursts
• physical deterioration: weight loss or diminished grooming

- other marked personality changes
- patient complaints about a physician's attitudes or demeanour

Signs of alcohol/substance abuse include:

- personality changes: increased anxiety, mood swings, decreased efficiency/reliability/decisiveness
- increased absenteeism
- increased reports of drug 'loss,' 'wastage,' or 'spoilage'
- visible intoxication on the job; alcohol on the breath
- individual insists on working alone
- individual insists on wearing long sleeves (to hide needle tracks) or disappears frequently (i.e., 'to the washroom')
- inappropriate affect/behaviour/comments

There are several ways of handling impaired colleagues. If they pose no immediate risk to themselves or to patients:

- State your concern in a gentle, private, and non-accusatory fashion. If possible, balance this with a positive comment ('You've always been a good physician, and I'm worried about you'). 'The non-coercive approach, with the possibility of punishment or coercion in the background, has been shown most successful.'[10]
- State your personal observations and those of others, so that denial can be reduced.
- Ask their view of the problem.
- Give them information on how to contact residents' professional associations that provide confidential help and ask them to tell you later what they have done. Offer to arrange an evaluation with a caregiver; do not take on the treatment yourself.
- Warn them that if you do not receive any feedback, or if the problem worsens, you will be obliged to discuss the matter confidentially with your residency director. (You may wish to do this first if you feel unable to confront the resident yourself.) Policies about reporting impaired physicians vary; reporting may be obligatory in your area.
- Point out that obtaining help does not have to result in suspension, loss of income, or expensive treatment, but that delay might.

If they pose an immediate risk to themselves:

- Accompany them to the emergency department or call the psychiatrist on duty in your hospital. Do not leave them alone. Consider calling your provincial or state residents' association hotline where available.

- If they pose an immediate risk to patients (e.g., are intoxicated before a delivery or a shift in the operating room or emergency department):
- Confront them discreetly with their current inability to perform. Offer to cover for them or to find coverage through the chief resident. If they refuse, call your attending physician immediately and inform your residency director. Patient safety is your priority.

Fortunately, programs like the JFK Family Practice Residency at the Robert Wood Johnson Medical School have written of their successes in working with impaired residents, demonstrating that intervention is well worth the effort. Consult the article by Winter and Birnberg[11] for a helpful algorithm on graded interventions that has proved helpful in such cases. (See the Resources at the end of this chapter for treatment/ referral information.)

STUDENTS

All physicians remember particularly good or bad residents in their training whose actions and characteristics strongly influenced their choice of specialties. Being role models and teachers for students adds a further stress to residents' professional lives. No one has taught them how to teach, so they must learn by doing and from observing good and bad examples. Interviews conducted by this author with residents indicate that a good resident teacher.

- 'provided orientation when we arrived'
- is accessible physically ('answers pages quickly') and emotionally ('doesn't make you feel stupid')
- has a good sense of humour and a capacity for making learning fun ('not overly anxious or compulsive')
- is efficient ('keeps rounds short') and punctual
- is practical ('simplifies things,' 'avoids esoteric emphasis')
- frequently gives positive feedback and patiently points out errors in patient care
- stands up to the attending physician when necessary ('makes own decisions')
- appears caring and conscientious and has good relations with patients and nurses
- is fair (e.g., 'about call duty')
- is available for one-on-one teaching
- knows how to handle team or interdisciplinary conflicts
- does not foster excessive competition

- is open to feedback him or herself
- delegates responsibility appropriately
- demonstrates appropriate use of investigations/consultation
- carries her or his own share of the workload
- remembers what it was like to be a student or junior
- creates a relaxed environment
- is willing to teach hands-on procedures and assign level-appropriate tasks (Read Edwards JC, Marier RL: *Clinical Teaching for Medical Residents: Roles, Techniques and Programs* [Springer Publishing, New York, 1988] to learn more about your role as a teacher. See also Morrison EH: Yesterday a learner, today a teacher too. *Pediatrics* 2000; 105: 235–243.)
- Remember to take your role as teacher seriously. Queen's University in Canada has produced guidelines for ethical teaching, excerpted below, which will help you reflect on your role as a teacher and may help launch discussion among residents and attending staff.

GUIDE TO THE ETHICAL BEHAVIOUR OF CLINICAL TEACHERS

Principles of Ethical Behaviour for all clinical teachers, including those who may not be engaged directly in clinical practice.

    I Consider first the well-being of the patient.
    II Honour your profession and its traditions.
    III Recognize your limitations and the special skills of others in the prevention and treatment of disease.
    IV Protect the patient's secrets (confidences).
    V Teach and be taught.
    VI Remember that integrity and professional ability should be your best advertisement.
    VII Be responsible in setting a value on your services.

RESPONSIBILITIES TO STUDENTS*

The ethical clinical teacher:

50. will treat students with respect regardless of level of training, race, creed, colour, gender, sexual orientation, or field of study;

51. will teach the knowledge, skills, attitudes and behaviour, and provide the experience that the student requires to become a physician in his/her chosen career;
52. will supervise students at all levels of training as appropriate to their knowledge, skills and experience;
53. will support and encourage students in their endeavours to learn and to develop their skills and attitudes and a sense of enquiry;
54. will allow responsibility commensurate with ability;
55. will see patients when so requested by students;
56. will teach to students the rationale for decisions, the reasons for conclusions, the reasoning behind investigation and treatment;
57. will discuss alternate diagnoses, investigations and therapeutic choices and the merits and risks of these;
58. will assess carefully and accurately students' abilities and provide prompt verbal and written feedback;
59. will assess only performance and not allow this assessment to be coloured by personal interactions;
60. will provide remedial teaching when so indicated by assessment;
61. will maintain a professional teacher–student relationship at all times and avoid the development of emotional, sexual, financial or other relationships with students;
62. will strive to conduct herself/himself in a fashion to be an excellent role model for students;
63. will refrain from addressing students in a disparaging fashion;
64. will refrain from intimidating or attempting to intimidate students;
65. will refrain from harassment of students in any fashion – emotional, physical or sexual.

*'Student' means any person involved in undergraduate or postgraduate health care training.

Reprinted with permission of R.D. Wigle and E.E. Eisenhauer, Queen's University

NURSING AND SUPPORT STAFF

Good relationships with nursing and other staff can make or break a residency experience, given a resident's high daily level of contact with them. The resident who feels threatened by competent nurses or physicians' assistants, and who feels superior or is sexist in interactions will be labelled early in training and will find it difficult to achieve the level of teamwork and camaraderie needed in the modern treating context.

To facilitate a good working relationship with nursing and other support staff:

- Introduce yourself to all the nurses on your service when you begin to work there. If you find it congenial, give them permission to use your first name. Remember their names as well.
- Ask them for their opinions and take their suggestions seriously. They may know the patient better than you do.
- Respect ward protocol and routines about orders, scheduling tests, and so on.
- Admit errors, including your own, and point out nursing errors in a private, non-accusatory, non-humiliating way.
- Do not show off or pull rank. Remember, you are working with fellow professionals.
- Do not bluff if you do not know something. Say that you will find out.
- Use appropriate humour. Avoid sexist or flirtatious remarks and behaviour.
- Try to develop a rapport with the head nurse, who may be a source of teaching and resource information and support.
- Be courteous and polite; say please and thank you.
- Keep disputes patient-oriented; do not let them become personal.

ATTENDING PHYSICIANS

Residents are in a unique and sometimes awkward position because they are hospital employees, student apprentices, and responsible physicians all at the same time. The attending physician ('staffman') is both a type of boss who does not pay or hire residents and a teacher who evaluates residents' performance and has considerable power over their future. Overall, clinical skills, personality, and teaching ability are what residents identify as factors in selecting a staff physician as a role model. A recent study shows that five types of issues affect the relationship between supervisor and trainee: compatibility of goals, communcation and feedback, power and rivalry, support and collegiality, and level of expertise of both parties.[12] Attending physicians vary in their approaches, just as senior residents do; some have an interest in teaching and interacting with their housestaff, whereas others are remote or absent, and merely bill for residents' services. The concept of 'medical student abuse' (either emotional or physical and sexual) applies equally to residents, who are particularly vulnerable because they need good evaluations to finish their training.

SIGNS OF TROUBLE IN RESIDENT–ATTENDING PHYSICIAN RELATIONSHIP

- sarcasm, harsh or hurtful criticism, verbal abuse, scapegoating (the target is usually a resident, who may complain covertly)
- lack of positive feedback
- racist, sexist, or other negative personal remarks directed at a resident
- physical abuse (e.g., scalpel throwing, sexual advances)
- decreased availability of the attending physician (late or absent for supervision, teaching, or rounds)
- covering up attending physician's mistakes or unethical behaviour
- increased resident anxiety in the context of supervision by the attending physician
- perception of the attending physician as incompetent, impaired, or unjust
- feeling that evaluations are unfair
- ceasing to care about work ('decathecting') because of an inability to please the attending physician

---

Dealing with the Problems

- Try to express your concerns privately to the attending physician.
- If you need to discuss your concerns with others, confide carefully and selectively to avoid gossip.
- Do not expose confidential issues in rounds or in front of colleagues.
- If you are acutely upset, excuse yourself briefly. Retain your compo-

sure, dignity, and professionalism. Do not retaliate and thereby lose your credibility.
- Document incidents, noting witnesses if necessary.
- Do not sign an evaluation you think is unfair. If you disagree with it, appeal the evaluation according to established procedures.
- If you are injured or sexually harassed, check your contract and report the incident to the residency program director and consider legal action.
- If these measures do not resolve the problem, consult the residency program director about mediation or change of service or hospital.
- If there is still no resolution, contact the following (according to the increasing severity of the problem): the university department head and/or the director of postgraduate education; the university harassment officer; the housestaff union lawyer; or the Resident Representative Committees at the Royal College of Physicians and Surgeons of Canada or the AMA.

PATIENTS

Although the relationship with the patient is central to medicine, it may be the most neglected area of learning in residency training. In actuality most residents spend only 20 per cent of their time actually interacting with patients. During training, personal discomfort, fatigue, time pressures, and team conflicts often erode this relationship to the point where residents become numb to the emotional needs of patients. This increased emotional buffering or distancing from patients and their suffering is the least adaptive and most damaging strategy used by residents to decrease personal levels of stress. It is a form of denial that precludes a unique possibility for supervised learning and for exploration of painful issues in care. Although technical medical care may be provided, no holistic healing takes place.

The growing emphasis on profit-driven, managed, and 'high-tech' care may prevent residents from developing primary-care, 'real world' skills, from being exposed to a wide range of socio-economic and health-related problems, and from providing continuity of care. One U.S. study surveying practising internal medicine graduates showed that only 42 per cent were 'fully satisfied' with their outpatient/primary-care training.

Physicians who stop caring have low career satisfaction levels, more lawsuits, and difficulty establishing practices. What is more insidious and disturbing, when empathy disappears from work it also disappears from life at home with one's partner, children, and friends.

Some patients are indeed difficult, argumentative, demanding, or angry. Others are so ill or upsetting to our wish to cure that we avoid them. Some reawaken our conflicts with parents and siblings and leave us bewildered at our response. Others simply happen to be number 32 of 70 in a busy emergency shift. Yet residents who do not learn to maintain empathy in the face of such stress compromise their present and future ability to truly heal their patients.

SIGNS OF TROUBLE IN RELATIONSHIPS WITH PATIENTS

- lack of emotional response to tragedy; rote functioning without affect
- increased anger towards patients manifested by rudeness, infantilization, and racist, sexist, ageist, or other disparaging or attempted humorous remarks
- identification of patients by body part, disease, or room number
- tendency to blame patients for illnesses or for physician-patient stalemates
- rushed or perfunctory interviews; failure to obtain personal and social histories of patients
- fantasies of a 'problem patient's' death or moving away
- increased authoritarian style or attempt to force treatment options or religious views on patients
- denial of patient's illness or pathologic features despite evidence
- emotional overinvolvement or overidentification with patients (including sexual behaviour; see guidelines regarding boundary violations)
- avoidant behaviour with certain patients
- hiding behind the anonymity of rounds (i.e., not providing your name to the patient)
- increased tendency to refer patients on, rather than to deal with difficulties directly

---

Avoiding Boundary Violations[13]

The following guidelines suggest approaches for avoiding complaints of sexual misconduct and preventing boundary violations:

1. Avoid any behaviour, gestures, or expressions that may be seductive or sexually demeaning to a patient.
2. Show sensitivity and respect for the patient's privacy and comfort at all times:
   - do not watch a patient dress or undress
   - provide privacy and appropriate covers and gowns
   - knock before entering the room.
3. Obtain permission to do intimate examinations, offer explanations as to the necessity of the examination, and answer anticipated questions concerning the examination.
4. Use gloves when examining genitals.
5. Do not make sexualized comments about a patient's body or clothing.
6. Do not make sexualized or sexually demeaning comments to a patient.
7. Do not criticize a patient's sexual orientation.
8. Do not ask or make comments about potential sexual performance except where the examination or consultation is pertinent to the issue of sexual function or dysfunction.
9. Do not ask details of sexual history or sexual likes/dislikes unless related to the purpose of the consultation or examination.
10. Do not request a date with a patient.
11. Do not kiss a patient. Do offer appropriate supportive contact when warranted.
12. Do not engage in any contact that is sexual (from touching to intercourse).
13. Do not talk about your own sexual preferences, fantasies, problems, activities, or performance.
14. Learn to detect and deflect seductive patients and to control the therapeutic setting.
15. Maintain good records which indicate the necessity for intimate examinations or questions of a sexual nature as well as the pertinent positive or negative clinical findings.
16. Patients have the right to have a third party present during internal/intimate examinations if they wish, with the exception of life-threatening emergencies. In some cases, the physician will be able to provide this third party. In cases where the physician is unable to provide such a person, patients should be informed that they may bring a person of their choosing with them. In non-emergency situations, physicians have the right to insist that a third party be present during internal/intimate examinations, and to refuse to conduct this

examination if the patient refuses consent for a third party to be in the room.

Avoiding/Dealing with Doctor–Patient Communication Problems[14]

- Empathy can be nurtured as well as compromised. Recognize under what circumstances it might be absent in you (e.g., overbooked clinics) and try to change what you can. A recent article in *JAMA* tracked mood states, interpersonal reactivity, and empathy over over the internship year and demonstrated a decline in trainee empathy over that period.[15] Don't let this happen to you.
- Recognize whether patients of a certain age or type repeatedly produce intense feelings in you (e.g., anger, lust, or sorrow) and try to determine whether they have hit a nerve in you ('counter-transference') or whether they are projecting their feelings on to you to give you a taste of their negative experience.
- Pay more attention to the patient's experience and less to your own performance anxiety, which will diminish with clinical experience.
- Distinguish your or your patient's anger at the system from your anger with each other so that it does not contaminate your interaction. Agreeing with a patient's upset will make you an ally rather than an adversary and may defuse conflict.
- Keep a record or journal of your emotional responses to key residency developmental or 'initiation' issues – for example, the first death of a patient (see below), first delivery, first bearing of bad news – and refer to it when you are feeling emotionally numb.

DELIVERING BAD NEWS[16]

- Bad news is best delivered when you have time for the patient. Make sure that you and the patient are reasonably comfortable; sit down. A pleasant room and private setting are extremely helpful.
- Watch patients for all-important non-verbal cues as to how they are listening to you. Be prepared for strong emotions and acknowledge them.
- Straightforwardness and lack of prevarication are essential.
- Keep medical terms to a minimum.
- Give patients the chance to be prepared for what you say: give

them a warning that you are about to tell them something very difficult.

- Patients must be given time to express their fears and worries. They will need to understand the news in their own terms and realize how it is likely to affect their future.
- Be well prepared for the session: try to have a plan for disclosure before the interview, be as informed as possible about the patient's problem, and know how to get answers for the patient if you cannot answer his or her questions. Know what the patient needs to do next.
- Be available and schedule a follow-up session even if you are about to refer the patient to a specialist. Patients will appreciate your ongoing concern.
- Do not be surprised if you are more worked up about the news than the patient is. Patients can show true resilience or complete denial in the face of seemingly disastrous news.

Other Tips to Enhance Communication with Your Patient

- Do not expect the same level of stoicism from patients that you expect from yourself. Learn to recognize cultural and personality- and more traditional sex-related differences in the expression of pain, anger, and grief.
- Make a point of chatting with your patients and try to learn at least one fact about their lives that will make them more human to you (e.g., the man with dementia on 8D used to be a composer).
- Let positive counter-transference happen consciously and selectively (e.g., 'that old lady in the emergency department hallway could be my grandmother').
- Remember your own experiences of illness, loss, discomfort, and vulnerability. These may differ from those of your patients, but the memory will help to link you in understanding.
- Do not be afraid to let your patients express their emotions. If you are afraid, find out why in therapy, in supervision, or in a resident support or Balint-style group rather than refer the patients for psychiatric treatment. When appropriate, consider acknowledging your feelings to your patient (e.g., 'I am tired today because I was on duty all night').
- Get to know your patient's family when possible, and try to be avail-

able for brief education sessions. This may help your patient cooperate with your treatment, which will diminish your workload.

- Identify your patients' psychosocial needs. After you have done the groundwork, you may want to recruit help from the departments of psychology or psychiatry, social work, and chaplaincy. But do not call them in simply because you do not want to deal with these needs. You must not dilute your responsibility to your patients.
- Study your referral patterns to see whether you avoid certain problems with patients.
- Keep informed about key psychosocial issues, which often manifest themselves in patients if you take the trouble to ask.
- Be sensitive to the patient's feelings of being undressed or exposed. Knock before entering a room.
- Maintain good eye contact with the patient; avoid taking excessive notes.
- Ask how the patient would like to be addressed (first name/title) and make sure he or she knows *your* name.
- Try to sit or stand at the same level as the patient so as not to be intimidating.
- Increase cross-cultural awareness by asking about your patient's background, learning of new language skills, and reading. Where appropriate, use a reliable family member or professional translator.
- Don't get angry about non-compliance with medication or treatment. Explore the patient's fears, misconceptions, side-effects, and financial worries (re: drug cost) instead.
- Use open-ended questions and don't interrupt.
- Ask the patient about fantasies ('What do *you* think it is?'), feelings, fears, and expectations about the illness.
- Make your explanations short, clear, and concise. Don't use jargon. Provide printed material if available.
- *Negotiate*, rather than dictate, management and the treatment plan with the patient, as an authoritarian stance may lower compliance.
- Offer the patient and his/her family self-help group information for added support. Two U.S. Clearing House Hotlines which will direct requests are the National Health Information Center (1-800-336-4797) and the New Jersey Self-Help Clearing House (1-800-367-6274).
- Try to follow your patients right through their illness. You'll learn much more through offering continuity of care in both the inpatient and outpatient setting.

- Be open to patient's wish to explore alternative forms of healing (like acupuncture or herbal medicine) as an adjunct to conventional care, if it enhances his or her sense of control and self-care. To learn more, check out this Website: http://www.yahoo.com/health/alternative_medicine

Remaining Sensitive and Compassionate about Death

Residents frequently report that, although they are often called to confirm the death of a patient, they receive no guidelines on how to do so from a compassionate as well as a medicolegal point of view. It makes sense to request seminars on death and dying, as they have been shown to increase levels of confidence and empathy in residents caring for the dying.[17] (Check out www.epec.net for a CME program called Education for Physicians on End of Life Care by Dr Linda Emanuel.)

Death is confirmed by

- dilated, fixed pupils
- no carotid pulse
- no heart sounds and breath sounds for over one minute.

When you have confirmed a death:

1. Take a quiet moment to acknowledge this patient's life and passage. Remember that it is an honour to be involved at the time of death of a human being, not a nuisance.
2. If family members are present express, your condolences in an unrushed fashion. (During your training, learn all you can about culturally different interpretations of death, burial, and mourning so that you can be sensitive with patients' families around the death of their loved one).
3. If the family are not present, speak to ward nurses who knew the patient about the best way to contact the patient's family. If appropriate, notify the staff physician supervising care, who may wish to make the call. If you call the family, identify yourself and ask for the next of kin. State at what time the patient died and whether or not you were directly involved in his or her care. Ask if the person would like to come in to be with the body, and notify the nurses of that decision. Reassure the family member that the individual died peacefully, with good nursing care.
4. Record in the patient's chart the date and time you were called and the above clinical data regarding confirmation of death.

> **SAMPLE CHARTING**
>
> Called to pronounce death of Mrs X. Patient was unresponsive to verbal/tactile stimulus. Pupils were fixed/dilated. No breath/heart sounds heard. No carotid pulse felt. Patient pronounced dead at 23:42, 6 Nov. 2003.

5. The death certificate is usually completed the next day. Find out local regulations regarding signing the death certificate, i.e., to distinguish coroner versus non-coroner cases. Speak to your chief resident or attending physician if in doubt.
6. If a clinical autopsy or postmortem is medically indicated, clarify the reasons with your attending staff / treatment team and seek written permission in a sensitive fashion from the next of kin or executor of the estate. Explain to the next of kin that an autopsy may prove useful in better understanding the patient's disease, but that family wishes will be respected.

Learning beyond Your Specialty

No matter what your specialty, increasing your knowledge of psychosocial issues can only help you provide better care. Consult an up-to-date psychiatric or behavioural medicine textbook or do a medline search on the following topics. Incorporate these into rounds, teaching, and case management. Invite guest consultants to discuss them as well. Modules on several of these topics may be found at www.amsa.org.

Topics Related to Psychosocial Issues

Alcohol and substance abuse
Alternative therapies
Anxiety
Attention deficit, enuresis, and other childhood problems
Brief psychotherapy
Child and sexual abuse
Compliance/non-compliance with treatment
Corrections facilities / prison health care
Cost-benefit decision analysis
Cultural aspects of care

Death and dying
Dementia
Depression and bipolar disorder
'Difficult' patients
Disability and disability-insurance protocols
The doctor–patient relationship
Drug abuse
Eating disorders
Empathy
End-of-life care/decisions
Epidemiology
Ethical issues in care including euthanasia, physician-assisted suicide
Family violence
Gay/lesbian, bisexual, and transgendered health issues
Gender issues in medical care
Geriatric care
Grief and mourning
HIV-AIDS – medical and psychosocial care
Illness behaviour
Insomnia
Life-cycle issues
Medicare
Multiculturalism
Narrative in medicine
Obsessive-compulsive disorders
Occupational health
Pain diagnosis and management
Palliative care
Personality disorders
Phobias
Prayer and healing
Pregnancy
Prevention (Health)
Psychiatric emergencies
Psychiatry and medicine
Psychogeriatrics
Rural medicine
Schizophrenia
Sexual assault
Sexual dysfunction

Smoking cessation
Spousal abuse (male and female)
Stress management
Suicide
Women's health and health research

Literature and Medicine

As well as familiarizing yourself with updated psychosocial articles, consider the use of literary classics for learning as these can facilitate individual reflection and group discussion on ethical issues of care and or human relationships. They can also innoculate you against cynicism about the profession. Check out journals of medicine and the humanities like ARS MEDICA (www.mtsinai.on.ca/arsmedica) or the *Bellevue Literary Review* (www.blreview.org).

Here is a list from the 'Great Books in Medical Ethics' course offered by the Evanston (IL) Hospital Department of Medicine:

The Doctor's Dilemma – George Bernard Shaw
The Hippocratic Oath
Cancer Ward – Alexander Solzhenitsyn
The Death of Ivan Illych – Leo Tolstoy
An Enemy of the People – Henrik Ibsen
A Very Easy Death – Simone De Beauvoir
The Plague – Albert Camus
'A Country Doctor' (story) – Franz Kafka
'Ward Six' (story) – Anton Chekhov
Tender Is the Night – F. Scott Fitzgerald
Frankenstein – Mary Shelley
Erewhon – Samuel Butler
The Power and the Glory – Graham Greene
The Imaginary Invalid and *The Doctor in Spite of Himself* – Molière
Man's Search for Meaning – Victor Frankl
The Elephant Man – Bernard Pomeranz
The Physician in Literature (excerpts) – Norman Cousins
Equus – Peter Shaffer

Forty-two Classic Films/videos to Facilitate Group Discussion of Physician Identity and the Doctor–Patient Relationship

1. *And the Band Played On*
2. *Article 99*

3. *Awakenings*
4. *Breaking the Waves*
5. *Celebration (Festen)*
6. *The Citadel*
7. *Cleo from 5:00–7:00*
8. *Common Threads: Stories from the AIDS Quilt*
9. *Dancer in the Dark*
10. *Death of a Salesman*
11. *Death Takes a Holiday*
12. *The Doctor*
13. *The Elephant Man*
14. *Frances*
15. *Happiness*
16. *Hospital*
17. *Ikira*
18. *I Never Promised You a Rose Garden*
19. *Kingdom*
20. *The Last Angry Man*
21. *Lorenzo's Oil*
22. *The Lost Weekend*
23. *Magnificent Obsession*
24. *Magnolia*
25. *Marnie*
26. *M*A*S*H*
27. *Murmur of the Heart*
28. *My Left Foot*
29. *One Flew Over the Cuckoo's Nest*
30. *Ordinary People*
31. *Philadelphia*
32. *The Prince of Tides*
33. *Resurrection*
34. *Scenes from Silver Lake*
35. *The Snake Pit*
36. *Spellbound*
37. *Sunday Bloody Sunday*
38. *Sybil*
39. *Terms of Endearment*
40. *White Corridors*
41. *Whose Life Is It Anyway?*
42. *Wild Strawberries*

REFERENCES

1 Landau C, Hall S, Wartman SA et al: Stress in social and family relationships during the medical residency. *J Med Educ* 1986; 61: 654–660

2 Smith MF, Andrasik F, Quinn SJ: Stressors and psychological symptoms of family practice residents and spouses. *J Med Educ* 1988; 63: 397–405

3 Myers M: *Doctors' Marriages: A Look at the Problems and Their Solutions.* Plenum Med Bks, New York, 1988

4 Guldner GT: Long-distance relationships and emergency medicine residency. *Ann Emerg Med* 2001; 37(1): 103–106

5 Jaco JM: *Can We Live with This Job?* PAIRO, Toronto, 1989

6 Adapted from La Puma J, Preist E: Is there a doctor in the house? An analysis of the practice of physicians treating their own families. *JAMA* 1992; 267(3): 1810–1812

7 Dempsey L, Ecker J: Understanding the dating guidelines. *CPSO Members' Dialogues* Nov 1994; 9–11

8 Jellinek MS: Recognition and management of discord within housestaff teams. *JAMA* 1985; 256: 754–755

9 Adapted from Goldman L, Lee T, Rudd P: Ten commandments for effective consultation. *Arch Intern Med* 1983; 143: 1753–1755

10 Tokarz JP, Bremer W, Peter K: *Beyond Survival: A Book Prepared by and for Resident Physicians to Meet the Challenge of the Impaired Physician and to Promote Well-Being through Medical Education.* Am Med Assoc, Chicago, 1979

11 Winter RO, Birnberg B: Working with impaired residents: trials, tribulations, and successes. *Fam Med* 2002; 34(3): 190–196.

12 Sinai J, Tiberius RG, de Groot J, Brunet A, Voore P: Developing a training program to improve supervisor–resident relationships, step 1: defining the types of issues. *Teach Learn Med* 2001; 13(2): 80–85.

13 Reprinted with permission from *Members' Dialogue* (CPSO), Nov 1993

14 Peterkin AD: Encouraging empathy. *Curr Ther* (*Med Post Suppl*) Sept 1989; 6, 8, 34

15 Bellini LM, Baime M, Shea JA: Variation of mood and empathy during internship. *JAMA* 2002; 287(23): 3143–3146

16 Reprinted with permission from Hébert P: *Doing It Right: A Practical Guide to Ethics for Physicians and Medical Trainees.* Oxford Univ Pr, Don Mills, ON, 1996. See also Ptacek JT, Eberhardt T: Breaking bad news: a review of the literature. *JAMA* 1996; 276: 496–502

17 Bagatell R, Meyer R, Herron S, Berger A, Villar R: When children die: a seminar series for pediatric residents. *Pediatrics* 2002; 110(2 pt 1): 348–353

OTHER REFERENCES

Campo R: *The Healing Art: A Doctor's Black Bag of Poetry*. W.W. Norton, New York, 2003

Cassell EJ: *The Nature of Suffering and the Goals of Medicine*. Oxford Univ Pr, New York, 1991

Pierce L: *The Patient–Physician Relationship: A Literature Review*. Canadian Medical Association, Ottawa, 1994

Roter DL, Hall JL: *Doctors Talking with Patient / Patients Talking with Doctors: Improving Communication in Clinical Visits*. Auburn House, Westport, CT, 1992

Spiro H. et al.: *Empathy and the Practise of Medicine: Beyond Pills and the Scalpel*. Yale Univ P, New Haven, 1996

RESOURCES FOR HELP WITH SUBSTANCE ABUSE

Aid for Impaired Medical Students program, University of Tennessee Health Science Center, Coleman College of Medicine

American Medical Association. (312) 464–5066

American Medical Student Association. Email: dsp@www.amsa.org

American Society of Addiction Medicine. www.asam.org

CAIR (Canadian Association of Interns and Residents' Resident Wellbeing Committee). www.cair.ca – cair@magma.ca

Center for Substance Abuse Treatment. 1-800-622–HELP

Coombs RH: *Drug-impaired Professionals: How Physicians, Dentists, Pharmacists, Nurses, Attorneys, and Airline Pilots Get Into and Out of Addiction*. Harvard Univ Pr, Cambridge, MA, 1997

National Clearinghouse for Alcohol and Drug Information. 1-800-729-6686.

National Institute on Drug Abuse. www.nida.nih.gov

Ontario Medical Association Physician Health Program. 1-800-267-6973. www.oma.org

Substance Abuse and Mental Health Services Administration. www.samhsa.gov

Talbott Recovery Campus. www.talbottcampus.com

(from Payne AM: Doctors in distress. *The New Physician* 2001; May–June: 19–23)

6. *Unique Concerns*

WOMEN

Back in 1989, when the first edition of this book came out, 44 per cent of Canadian medical school graduates were women, compared with 6 per cent in 1959 and 33 per cent in 1981. In 1990, 30 per cent of all residents in the United States were women; by the year 2010 it is predicted that well over half of all U.S. physicians will be women.[1] In 2003 the number of women enrolled in medical school surpassed 50 per cent in many provinces in Canada. In 1977 women were not represented in one-third of specialties.[2] In most countries, women tend to choose primary care fields for specialization: internal medicine, pediatrics, obstetrics, gynecology, family practice, and psychiatry. Several studies show that in residency women tend to work more hours, experience more stress, and report more personal, emotional, and relationship problems than do their male counterparts.[3] They have a higher debt load on graduating and tend to earn less money in practice than men.

On the other hand, women have been shown to have similar academic but better communication skills, and to experience fewer lawsuits and higher levels of career satisfaction than men.[4] (Some of these findings may be attributable to the fact that women show more candour in surveys on residency stress or may be more open to seeking help.) It is, however, important to recognize some of the unique pressures women face during their medical careers that men do not experience, or may experience to a lesser degree.

Medicine in North America has been and continues to be a male-dominated field to which women have been obliged to adapt. Women residents have few female role models among teachers and administrators in their chosen career, and only sometimes find the satisfying mentoring that all developing physicians require. Women in medicine experience what has been called 'role strain,' in that they are expected to conform simultaneously to cultural stereotypes of the feminine 'caregiver' who will humanize a harsh medical technology and of the competent, competitive physician. Their hectic schedules often wreak havoc with the expectations they and others have of their capacity to manage the responsibilities of housekeeping, parenting, and supporting family members.

In the hospital setting, women nurses sometimes compete with or are less tolerant of women physicians. Colleagues may expect them to carry a higher female or pediatric patient load, and patients may doubt their credibility or not address them as 'doctor.' Sexual harassment by colleagues and patients is also a more serious problem for women residents than for men. In a sample of 599 female doctors, 77 per cent reported being sexually harassed by patients at least once since becoming physicians (see chapter 1). Pregnancy and issues related to the timing of a family pose logistic and personal dilemmas for couples. An AMA study found that one-half of women physicians who had children had had their first, and one-quarter had had their second, child during residency.[5] Despite these facts, many U.S. schools and programs still do not have formal maternity-leave policies. A recent study showed that in U.S. Obs-Gyn programs only 80 per cent had maternity leaves and 69 per cent paternity leaves. And they are in the business of delivering babies![6] In Canada, maternity benefits are in all residents' contracts, although the length of leave may vary from program to program. However, a pregnant resident may encounter subtle and not so subtle expressions of resentment from colleagues who believe they will have to carry her clinical load.[7]

Current Trends among Women in Medicine[3,8]

- By the year 2000, 35 per cent of all physicians in Canada were women.
- Within a decade of completing training, one-third of women physicians will take maternity leave, and 24 per cent prolonged leave for other reasons. Most will have shorter work weeks than their male counterparts.[9]
- Currently over 50 per cent of applicants to medical schools in Canada are women, compared with 48 per cent in the United States.[3]
- Only 75 of 2,000 chairpersons of U.S. medical school departments in

1990 were women (but currently 30 per cent of medical faculty members are women).[3]
- Two-thirds of practising women physicians in the United States have children.[3]

Suggestions for Women

- Apply to a residency program that has a significant or growing representation of women, particularly in leadership roles.
- Review contract issues on maternity leave and time-sharing options before applying.
- Make an effort to form links with women colleagues. If you encounter an attending physician or lecturer who appears to have managed juggling family and career life successfully, ask to keep in touch with her from time to time. Find a mentor.
- Consider forming a women's residency support group or lecture series. Nominate a person in your hospital as a contact person for women's issues or grievances. Include medical students.
- Investigate the services provided by the national and international medical women's groups. Here are some useful resources for assisting the process:
  - The American Medical Women's Association offers a Harassment and Gender Discrimination Resource and Information Phone Line for physicians and students. (703) 838-0500.
  - The *Journal of the American Medical Women's Association* publishes reports on gender discrimination and sexual harassment in medicine.
  - Consider contacting the American Medical Association, Women in Medicine Services, 515 North State Street, Chicago, IL 60610.
  - The address of the Equal Employment Opportunity Commission is 1801 L Street NW, Washington, DC 20507. 1-800-669-EEOC.
- Order these documents/publications:
  - Bownan M, Frank E, Allen D: *Women in Medicine: Career and Life Management.* Springer, New York, 2002
  - *Building a Stronger Women's Program: Enhancing the Educational and Professional Environment*, an Association of American Medical Colleges publication, Washington, 1993
  - The Council on Graduate Medical Education's Fifth Report to Congress, *Women and Medicine'* Spring 1995
  - *New and Emerging Issues*, a 1991 career-oriented video from the

Committee on Women in Family Medicine of the American Academy of Family Physicians (address: 8880 Ward Parkway, Kansas City MO 61114)

Pregnancy

- Where possible, plan carefully the timing of your pregnancy. Notify your residency program director of your dates so that together you can plan a reasonable schedule (i.e., lighter rotations before delivery).
- Be open with colleagues about dates and continuing difficulties. Do not become apologetic or overcompensating.
- Maintain close ties with your obstetrician or general practitioner in case you experience complications or need letters for sick leave or scheduling recommendations.
- Three months has been shown to be the minimum period that should be allotted for maternity leave to allow for adequate rest and reorganization and to take account of daycare regulations on the age at which infants are accepted. Cite the Sayres[7] paper if you have to negotiate the details of your maternity leave. As well, the CIR has prepared a highly recommended resource packet of union ideas/proposals/programs called *Pregnancy in Residency: A Union Perspective.* Plan carefully, and well in advance, the support you need with the logistics around your delivery and child care. (See the section on parenting in chapter 5 for further suggestions.)

INTERNATIONAL MEDICAL GRADUATES (IMGs)[9]

Historically there have been no more than 100 places for foreign medical graduates (IMGs) per year in Canadian residency programs, and the proportion of IMGs in U.S. residencies dropped from 20.2 per cent in 1979 to 15.3 per cent in 1988. Since the introduction of a clinical-skills assessment examination in 1998 for Educational Commission for Foreign Medical Graduates (ECFMG) certification, a drop in IMG applicants has been noted. The number of foreign-trained Americans applying for places in U.S. programs dropped as well during this period. Most international graduates have come from India, the Caribbean, Mexico, the Philippines, and Pakistan. In 1990, 18 per cent of all U.S. residency positions were filled by IMGs. Little has been written about the stresses particular to IMGs, but several of them are well known.

Not only do IMGs have to cope with the rigours of residency scheduling and high levels of responsibility, but they must also adjust to the medical hierarchy, to changed legal status as immigrants or refugees, and to a new country, culture, language, and ethical or religious system. Rules governing male–female dynamics may differ. Dress and personal hygiene codes may be more stringent or relaxed. Family members may become isolated from the new culture and thus more dependent psychologically and financially on the resident. Adjustment and adaptation to a new culture creates significant stress for anyone and results in culture shock.[10] The social isolation of foreign residents caused by the absence of family or their own sensitivity about cultural differences can put them at high risk.

Foreign-trained residents who have studied in centres equipped with less technology or fewer resources than those in North America may experience particular struggles over competence, whereas those who have come from settings similar to North American centres resent the assumption by some that they are less skilled. Many IMGs have been delayed – some for ten years or more– in being accepted for internship because of restrictions related to language, medical qualifying exams, and citizenship requirements. Some provinces and states impose restrictive contracts on IMGs that oblige them on completion of training to work for up to four years in an underserviced area. Increased remuneration for working peripherally may not compensate for the inconvenience to the physician and his or her family.

Many IMGs experience a marked status shift; the resident from a Third World country may become more wealthy and comfortable than ever before, whereas professors who must repeat all of their training to obtain accreditation are often devastated initially. Regional differences in patients' acceptance of visible minorities or of those who speak with an unfamiliar accent can be significant, and many IMGs experience hostile and racist reactions from the patients they are expected to treat.

North Americans who complete medical school abroad are not exempt from added strain during their residency. Though they return to a culture they have known, it has continued to evolve in their absence; indeed, they often return to a different medical system (e.g., the Mexican-trained resident who returns to American medicine). They may feel apologetic or inadequate for not having been accepted in a North American medical school or for having learned different or less technological protocols. Canadian-trained physicians who acquire residencies in the United States are often bewildered by non-socialized, non-universal medical care.

Suggestions for IMGs

- Apply to a residency program that has significant representation of or a special entry program for IMGs or refugees. Recent physician shortages in Canada have led to an increased number of positions.
- Determine any contractual or practice-related restrictions before accepting an internship. If necessary, consult a lawyer who can help you avoid being exploited.
- Form a support group of other IMGs to prepare for qualifying exams. For information on the ECFMG exams see www.ecfmg.org. You can also meet others in your situation at exam preparation courses such as those offered by the Stanley Kaplan Co.
- Seek a mentor who is also an IMG (perhaps someone from your own country or culture), or someone informed on IMG issues whom you can consult from time to time for advice and support.
- As you adapt to a new culture, maintain close social ties with your family and ethnic community. Attend organized events with your family. Explore your contract for information on religious-holiday protections.
- Guard against a tendency to be overcritical of yourself because what you know is different. Ask questions and be open, rather than apologetic, about protocol differences. Ask your senior resident for intermittent one-on-one attention if you are weak in a particular area. Point out how you can enrich your program through your knowledge of other cultures/languages.
- Contact the national and international medical ethnic groups and associations. Your union may also have special committees/initiatives related to IMG training. (See resources listed on p. 107.)

VISIBLE-MINORITY RESIDENTS

Special incentive programs for Native students in Canada and for black, Hispanic, and Native (aboriginal) students in the United States have produced a limited increase in their representation in the profession. These students sometimes encounter resentment in residency because frequently such programs are believed to constitute 'reverse discrimination or racism' – that is, they are seen to give preferential treatment, or even exclusive access to medical training, to the participants solely because of their ethnic background. Many of these residents experience a socio-economic and status shift, because they are more educated or

better paid than many of their family members but are less affluent than
or socio-economically remote from their white resident counterparts.
They may experience a unique kind of marginality that leaves them
feeling suspect, or like 'impostors,' both at home and at work.

Residents whose skin colour others perceive as similar (e.g., those
from a variety of Asian backgrounds) may be 'lumped together' in the
minds of patients and colleagues. As happens with IMGs, these residents
may encounter subtle assumptions or biases in patients, colleagues, and
support staff, sometimes in direct personal comments, sometimes in
having patients from 'their' presumed ethnic group referred to them.

RELIGIOUS RESIDENTS

Religiously observant or devout residents, whether Christian, Jewish,
Muslim, Buddhist, Sikh, Hindu, followers of a Native traditional way, or
others with strong spiritual convictions may experience dilemmas about
such matters as abortion, contraception, non-marital unions, and homosexuality when asked to carry out duties or confirm advice that they find
immoral, unethical, or otherwise in conflict with their values.

THE PRAYER OF MAIMONIDES

Almighty God! With infinite wisdom has thou shaped the body
of man. Ten thousand time ten thousand organs has thou put
within it that move in harmony and without ceasing to keep in
all its beauty the whole – the body, the envelope of the immortal
soul ...

To Man has thou given the wisdom to soothe his brother's suffering, to know his disorders, to extract what substances may
heal, to learn their powers, and prepare and use them suitably
for every ill ...

Inspire in me a love for my art and for thy creatures. Let no thirst
for profit or seeking for renown or admiration take away from
my calling ... Keep within me strength of body and of soul, ever
ready, with cheerfulness, to help and succour rich and poor,
good and bad, enemy as well as friend. In the sufferer let me see
only the human being ... If those should wish to improve and

instruct me who are wiser than I, let my soul gladly follow their guidance; for vast is the scope of our art ...

In all things let me be content, in all but the great science of my calling. Let the thought never arise that I have attained to enough knowledge, but vouchsafe to me ever the strength, the leisure and the eagerness to add to what I know. For art is great, and the mind of man ever growing.

Almighty God! In thy mercy thou has chosen me to watch beside life and death in thy creatures. I now go to the work of my calling. In its high duties sustain me, so that it may bring benefit to mankind, for nothing, not even the least can flourish without thy help.

Etziony ME: *The Physician's Creed: An Anthology of Medical Prayers, Oaths and Codes of Ethics Written and Recited by Medical Practitioners through the Ages.* CC Thomas, Springfield, IL, 1973: 29–30

MEDICINE AND ILLNESS

Honour the doctor for his services,
for the Lord created him.
His skill comes from the Most High,
and he is rewarded by kings.
The doctor's knowledge gives him high standing
and wins him the admiration of the great.
The Lord has created medicines from the earth,
and a sensible man will not disparage them.
Was it not a tree that sweetened water
and so disclosed its properties?
The Lord has imparted knowledge to men,
that by their use of his marvels he may win praise;
by using them the doctor relieves pain
and from them the pharmacist makes up his mixture.
There is no end to the works of the Lord,
who spreads health over the whole world.

My son, if you have an illness, do not neglect it,
but pray to the Lord, and he will heal you.
Renounce your faults, amend your ways, and cleanse your heart
   from all sin.
Bring a savoury offering and bring flour for a token
and pour oil on the sacrifice; be as generous as you can.
Then call in the doctor, for the Lord created him;
do not let him leave you, for you need him.
There may come a time when your recovery is in their hands;
then they too will pray to the Lord to give them success in
   relieving pain
and finding a cure to save their patient's life.
When a man has sinned against his Maker, let him put himself in
   the doctor's hands.

Jerusalem Bible, Eccles. 38:1–15

MAIMONIDES' CODE FOR PHYSICIANS

O god, may the love of my art actuate me at all times; may neither avarice, nor miserliness, nor the thirst for glory or a great reputation engage my mind, for, enemies of truth and philanthropy, they could easily deceive me and make me forgetful of my lofty aim of doing good to thy children. Endow me with strength of heart and mind, so that both may be ready to serve the rich and the poor, the good and the wicked, friend and enemy, and that I may never see in the patient anything else but a fellow creature in pain.

   If physicians more learned than I wish to counsel me, inspire me with confidence in and obedience toward the recognition of them, for the study of the science is great. It is not given to one alone to see all that others see. May I be moderate in everything except in the knowledge of this science; so far as it is concerned, may I be insatiable; grant me the strength and opportunity always to correct what I have acquired, always to extend its domain; for knowledge is boundless and the spirit of human kind can also extend infinitely, daily to enrich itself with new acquirements.

from *The Code of Maimonides*. Yale Univ Pr, New Haven, CT, 1949

Suggestions for Visible-Minority and Religious Residents

- Apply to a residency program with significant visible-minority representation or a religious affiliation.
- Consider or find a mentor with similar cultural or religious traditions so that you can share problem solving.
- Speak with the hospital ethicist or chaplain about the best way to make your views known and understood to colleagues and patients.
- Challenge generalizations and stereotyping calmly when you encounter them clinically. You are in a unique position to educate ethnocentric or non-religious physicians.
- Consider forming a support group with other residents whose background or tradition is similar to yours.
- Consider inviting speakers and holding seminars for the hospital at large on treating specific groups of patients. Offer to be a minority representative in your hospital.
- Although the system may encourage 'tokenism,' affirm your individuality and level of skill and resist the temptation to overcompensate or prove something.
- Contact resource groups for information on conferences, grants, minority research opportunities, and services.
- All residents should recognize that there is value in finding or rediscovering a spiritual or faith-related focus during the stresses and challenges of residency, as it can be an important source of sustenance and growth. Check out the following resources:
  - International Center for the Integration of Health and Spirituality (www.icihs.org)
  - Robert Wood Johnson Foundation (www.rwjf.org)

A PHYSICIAN'S PRAYER

Dear Lord, give skill to my hand, clear vision to my mind, kindness and sympathy to my heart. Give me singleness of purpose, strength to lift at least a part of the burden of my suffering fellow mortals and a true realization of the privilege that is mine. Take from my heart all guile and worldliness that with the simple faith of a child I may rely on thee.

Author Unknown

GAY AND LESBIAN RESIDENTS

Gay and lesbian residents, who make up an estimated 10 per cent of the resident population, not only face particular challenges in their daily lives but also must deal with a medical hierarchy that can at times be rigid and intolerant. Gay men and women historically have been an invisible, rejected minority, and those in most residency programs still find it necessary to hide their sexual identity from colleagues. This results in social isolation, stigmatization, and missed peer support about shared issues, such as couple relationships.

The gay resident's partner may experience increased isolation because of a reluctance of the resident to socialize with colleagues, which may produce added couple conflict. The gay resident lacks public role models who are comfortable with their own professional and sexual identities, and therefore may not find a mentor.

Gay residents can be victims of social or sexual harassment from superiors but may remain silent to protect their own identities. They may let homophobic remarks by patients and colleagues go unchecked for fear of disclosing their orientation and thereby attracting hostility or suspicion. Such situations result in much unresolved anger.

Gay residents working with children in pediatrics or psychiatry may experience particular stress or feel suspect because of the common and unfounded misconceptions that homosexuals may 'contaminate' or molest children. Those considering a career in psychiatry will often be asked about sexual orientation before they enter a residency and will be assumed to be heterosexual by the professors who supervise their psychotherapy. If they choose to apply to a psychoanalytic institute for further training they will likely be rejected, because many analysts still see homosexuality as an 'arrest' in psychic development.

Some residents report being refused to specific programs because of perceived homosexuality or HIV-positive status. The gay male resident in medicine or surgery may experience marked anxiety when treating patients with AIDS because of his own fear of the disease as a member of a hard-hit community or because he or his lover is HIV-seropositive. He may also be worried about meeting social contacts clinically or patients socially.

Finally, many men and women only start to come to grips with their gay identity during the years they spend in residency. Regrettably, training demands can delay such important discoveries and personal growth.

Suggestions for Gay and Lesbian Residents

- Contact the Gay and Lesbian Medical Association (GLMA), formerly the American Association of Physicians for Human Rights, and the local gay press for notices of meetings of gay health-provider organizations in your city. These groups are welcoming to bisexual and transgendered members as well. The address of the GLMA is: 459 Fulton Street, Suite 107, San Francisco, CA 94102 (www.glma.org).
- Choose a residency program in a city with an active and political gay life. Such a city will also have a higher visible percentage of gay physicians who can help you in your career and serve as role models.
- As you get to know other residents and interns you will gradually perceive whom you can tell about your life. Do not shut yourself off from possible peer support for you and your partner.
- Do not feel obliged to let homophobic remarks go unchecked. Respond firmly and calmly. Use the situation as an opportunity to educate.
- Resist any tendency to overcompensate because of being gay or lesbian. If you are having particular difficulties with reconciling your sexual and professional identities seek help in the form of psychotherapy.
- Remember that you are not obliged to answer questions pertaining to sexual orientation in residency applications or employment interviews. The choice is yours.
- Encourage your program to provide sensitive, appropriate training regarding care of gay and lesbian patients. A video called *Caring for Gay and Lesbian Patients* is available from the Canadian Psychiatric Association (1-613-234-2815), as well as a new clinical guide, *Caring for Lesbian and Gay People*, from the University of Toronto Press (see References, no. 11).

RESIDENTS WITH A DISABILITY OR CHRONIC ILLNESS

Residents who are blind, use wheelchairs, or have a chronic illness (such as diabetes, chronic pain, lupus, or asthma) experience increased stress as a result of their disability that may in turn be worsened by residency-related stress. Residents with a visible impairment may have to work harder to establish credibility with patients and to deal repeatedly with social awkwardness in patients and colleagues in a way that sometimes wears down a successful coping style. Colleagues, in particular, may try to be overhelpful or may be reluctant to acknowledge the disability. Precedents of residents with most disabilities (including blindness and quadraplegia) now exist, but program directors may still be worried about these residents' 'efficacy and suitability' for the specialty.

The resident who becomes seriously ill during residency must contend with issues of loss, pain, and uncertainty in addition to the stresses of residency.

Suggestions for Residents with a Disability or Chronic Illness

- Good support from family, other housestaff, and hospital support staff is essential. Calculate the help you need, such as navigation, elevator service, and special meals, and request it. Never ask someone junior to you to make decisions for you. Try to form particular ties with porters, orderlies, nurses and aides, mail carriers, and elevator operators, who will probably be glad to help.
- Discuss your disability or illness openly with your program director and chief resident so that they can help you develop strategies. Do not hide periods of illness from colleagues, as such stoicism may compromise your own and your patients' care.
- Maintain close links with your personal physician so that you can get quick follow-up, treatment, and letters for sick leave or change of duties if required.
- Some patients are comforted to learn that their physician is not omnipotent and shares the experience of illness. Avoid the tendency to overcompensate, to neglect your personal life, or to be a 'super-doctor' because of your disability, but remember that you may have something to teach your housestaff team about the experience of being a patient.

REFERENCES

1 Etzel SI, Egan RL, Shevrin MP: Graduate medical education in the United States. *JAMA* 1989; 262: 1029–1037
2 Young EG: Relationship of residents' emotional problems, coping behaviours and gender. *J Med Educ* 1987; 62: 642–650
3 Bickel JA: Women physicians: change agents or second-class citizens? *Humane Med* 1990; 6: 101–105
4 Borsellino M: Female MD time off the job creates uncertainty for manpower planners. *Med Post* 27 Mar 1990

5 Franco K: Conflicts associated with a physician's pregnancy. *Am J Psychiatry* 1983; 140: 902–904

6 Davis JL, Baillie S, Hodgson CS, Vontver L, Platt LD: Maternity leave: existing policies of obstetrics and gynecology residency programs. *Obstet Gynecol* 2001; 98(6): 1093–1098

7 Sayres MA, Wyshak G, Denterlein G: Pregnancy during residency. *New Engl J Med* 1986; 314: 419–423

8 Barzansky B: Educational programs in U.S. medical schools 2001–2002. *JAMA* 2002; 288(9): 1067–1072

9 Educational Commission for Foreign Medical Graduates (www.ecfmg.org)

10 Kaplan HD, Sadock BJ: *Comprehensive Textbook of Psychiatry*, 5th ed. Williams & Wilkins, Baltimore, 1989: 1412–1413

11 Peterkin AD, Risdon, C: *Caring for Lesbian and Gay People: A Clinical Guide.* Univ of Toronto Pr, Toronto, 2003

RESOURCES FOR IMGs

American Association of International Medical Graduates (www.aaimg.com)
American College of International Physicians (www.acip.org)
American College of Physicians–American Society of Internal Medicine (www.acponline.org/img)
American Medical Student Association–International Members Caucus (www.amsa.org/member/intlmbrs.cfm)

7. Ethics Issues and Legal Considerations

Residents often have concerns about the risks of litigation during or after their training, and understandably seek ways to protect themselves. Educators in medical ethics suggest that this focus is sadly misplaced and that residents should concentrate on learning ethical ways to preserve their relationships with patients and to act in their best interests. Because ethical and legal principles naturally overlap, it is generally assumed that the ethical physician should rarely be sued, although the application of the law to specific issues and case dilemmas can vary among provinces and states.

Most residents have taken courses and discussed ethics as undergraduates, but formal learning about ethics during residency varies considerably from program to program.[1] Because residents make decisions about ethics and physician–patient relationships daily, the lack of formal help or instruction in these areas can add further stress to resident life. Trainees face conflict when they try to respect patients' autonomy if they believe that their own is compromised. Residents whose views differ from those of their patients or who witness malpractice will experience dissonance and confusion. Ethical disagreements with attending physicians, particularly concerning overtreatment often are not voiced and this represents a significant stressor.[2]

This chapter is intended to sensitize you to ethics issues and legal considerations. It is by no means a comprehensive summary of the issues, nor does it offer legal directives.

ETHIC ISSUES

As summarized by Perkins[3] in his classic review article, the DeCamp Foundation recommends that, during postgraduate training, residents should acquire ethical skills related to:

- moral aspects of medical practice
- informed-consent process
- patient refusal of treatment
- management of the incompetent patient
- withholding of information
- confidentiality
- management of the patient with a poor prognosis
- management of medical resources

You should reflect on the following summary of views on these matters[4-8] during your training in any specialty, seeking supervision when appropriate.

Moral Aspects of Medical Practice

Residents often experience conflict between their wish to heal ('beneficence') and patients' wish for autonomy and self-determination. In addition, residents' views of illness and of cultural or moral issues may differ dramatically from those of patients. They must learn to recognize these inner conflicts and how they relate to the patient, and to ascertain, and then respect, the patient's wishes, rather than adopt an authoritarian, omnipotent stance. If residents cannot appreciate a patient's position, either they should say so, explaining what this may mean to their physician–patient contract, or they should help the patient find alternative care. They remain responsible for their patient's care until another physician is found.

Informed-Consent Process

Informed consent exists to protect the patient, not the hospital or the caregiver. It consists of three key elements:

1. Information must be provided to the patient about the treatment or procedure, its purpose, risk–benefit ratio, alternatives, and expected results. Pertinent details must not be withheld because of the physician's wish to obtain consent.
2. Comprehension by and competence of the patient must be assured. Facts must be explained in clear, everyday language with no jargon.
3. Consent must be voluntary – that is, the physician states his or her opinion or position but does not coerce the patient into making a decision. It is important to keep in mind that 'blanket consent' given by the patient on entering hospital is not sufficient. Consent must be sought and obtained for each new procedure or change in treatment.

Patient Refusal of Treatment

A patient has the right to refuse treatment if his or her reason is adequately explored and is not based solely on misunderstanding, misinformation (e.g., from physician-patient conflict), or coercion from external sources. The likely consequences of failure to give treatment should be presented to the patient. In most hospitals a patient is then asked to sign a statement affirming that treatment has been refused in full knowledge of these consequences. It is important to remember that this choice should not be equated with incompetence or a suicidal tendency in the patient, although these possibilities must be explored.

Management of the Incompetent Patient

Incompetent patients are unable to make decisions about their own care and well-being. They cannot understand information relevant to a decision, consider choices logically, make a choice consistent with their own values, or communicate that choice.[3] Most incompetent patients have chronic neurologic conditions that affect cognition, insight, and memory, such as dementia or post-stroke or post-traumatic syndromes. Legislation defining who can declare a patient incompetent varies; in some areas it is any physician, whereas in others it must be a psychiatrist. Chart documentation always includes a mental-status exam and a commentary on the three criteria for informed consent (information, comprehension, and voluntariness). Verify the appropriate procedure with the hospital's social services department.

If informed consent cannot be given because of incompetence, the resident, with the help of a social worker, will want to initiate the proceedings for 'curatorship' or 'guardianship,' the details and designations of which vary from province to province and from state to state. The 'proxy' or 'tutor' is an appointed person who must be able to determine what the patient would have wished if able to choose, not what is best for the estate, the family or the proxy. Ideally this person is someone who loves and respects the patient and may be a family member, but it cannot be assumed that the spouse or sibling will best serve the patient's interests.

Withholding Information

Physicians have traditionally used 'therapeutic privilege' to withhold potentially 'harmful' or 'devastating' information from a patient, often at the request of the family. Today this is seldom deemed appropriate by lawyers and ethics consultants because the competent patient has the right to know about diagnosis, treatment, prognosis, alternatives, and risks. As Perkins[3] has pointed out, the question is not *whether* to tell, but *how* to tell. The physician is ethically bound to convey difficult news compassionately and to deal with the results, while continually offering information and support to the patient.

Confidentiality

The resident should not release information about a patient to anyone without clear authorization or express approval, which should be documented in the chart. Caution with respect to protection of and access to medical records must be emphasized to all staff, especially with respect to new technologies such as computerized records, e-mail, fax machines, and cellular telephones which may be accessed by unauthorized individuals. 'Implied consent' traditionally referred to a physician divulging details of a case to family members or other members of the treatment team, but even this practice should be explored with the patient and recorded. Residents are often casual in the way they discuss certain patients with each other (i.e., in an elevator or in the cafeteria), because of the potential for learning involved or an unconscious need to vent their feelings. This practice is increasingly being viewed as unethical because it may violate a patient's consent about what is said about him or her, and to whom.

Exceptions to absolute protection of a patient's medical privacy vary locally, but include the following situations:

- a subpoena to give evidence in court (where files and documents can be held as evidence)
- a court order or search permit to produce a patient's chart (not simply a visit from a police officer or sheriff)
- reporting to appropriate authorities child or elder abuse, gunshot wounds, unsafe drivers and pilots, certain venereal diseases, and workplace accidents
- reporting to appropriate authorities a patient's likely harm to self or others (suicide, homicide, rape, kidnapping, violent behaviour, etc.)

Managing the Patient with a Poor Prognosis[9]

Every resident during training is faced with decisions about continuing treatment as opposed to palliation and non-resuscitation of terminally ill patients, and must become familiar with making such distinctions.

Guidelines from various medical, nursing, and hospital associations for non-resuscitation include the following:

- an assessment that the condition is irreversible and estimates of how long the patient might live without intervention, as well as of the consequence of no-code status (i.e, 'do not resuscitate' order)
- an assessment of the patient's competence and ability to understand risks, benefits, consequences, and options with respect to a no-code status
- consultation with an appropriate family member if the patient is incompetent
- documentation of the attending physician's approval and a second opinion from another physician or clinical ethics consultant if there is doubt about the suitability of a no-code status
- a clear order written in the chart to clarify the no-code status

Management of Medical Resources

The management of medical resources is a controversial issue beyond the scope of this discussion, and its ramifications differ considerably between socialized medical systems (as in Canada) and private ones (as in the United States, where the AMA has prepared a document called the 'AMA Ethical and Judicial Affairs Ethics Guidelines for Managed Care'). The resident should, however, remember the fundamental principle that every human being is entitled to appropriate care, regardless of diagnosis, race, creed, or ability to pay.

PATIENT–PHYSICIAN COVENANT

Medicine is, at its centre, a moral enterprise grounded in a covenant of trust. This covenant obliges physicians to be competent and to use their competence in the patient's best interests. Physicians, therefore, are both intellectually and morally obliged to act as advocates for the sick wherever their welfare is threatened and for their health at all times.

Today, this covenant of trust is significantly threatened. From within, there is growing legitimation of the physician's materialistic self-interest; from without, for-profit forces press the physician into the role of commercial agent to enhance the profitability of health care organizations. Such distortions of the physician's responsibility degrade the physician–patient relationship that is the central element and structure of clinical care. To capitulate to these alterations of the trust relationship is to significantly alter the physician's role as healer, carer, helper, and advocate for the sick and for the health of all.

By its traditions and very nature, medicine is a special kind of human activity – one that cannot be pursued effectively without the virtues of humility, honesty, intellectual integrity, compassion, and effacement of excessive self-interest. These traits mark physicians as members of a moral community dedicated to something other than its own self-interest.

Our first obligation must be to serve the good of those persons who seek our help and trust us to provide it. Physicians, as physicians, are not, and must never be, commercial entrepreneurs, gateclosers, or agents of fiscal policy that runs counter to our trust. Any defection from primacy of the patient's well-being places the patient at risk by treatment that may compromise quality of or access to medical care.

We believe the medical profession must reaffirm the primacy of its obligation to the patient through national, state, and local professional societies; our academic research, and hospital organizations; and especially through personal behaviour. As advocates for the promotion of health and support of the sick, we are called upon to discuss, defend, and promulgate medical care by every ethical means available. Only by caring and advocating for the patient can the integrity of our profession be affirmed. Thus we honour our covenant of trust with patients.

From Crawshaw R, Rogers DE, Pellegrino ED, Bulger RJ, Lundberg GD, Bristow LR, Cassel CK, Barondess JA: Patient–physician covenant. *JAMA* 1995; 273(19): 1553. Reprinted with permission

Learning More about Ethical Issues

The following suggestions are offered for learning more about medical ethics.

- Request and attend ethics case conferences, grand rounds, lectures, and retreats.
- Try to incorporate ethics concerns into your regular case presentations or into other residents' discussion groups to stimulate discussion.
- Seek guidance and examples from more senior residents and attending physicians.
- Contact the hospital's ethics consultant about the particular difficulties of a case.
- Pay attention to your own levels of discomfort when you sense something is unethical, and try to discuss these feelings with a colleague. Do not dismiss them or let them add to your anxiety.
- Consult the books by Jonsen[4] and Beauchamp[5] in the References; they are practical, case-oriented pocket guides to medical ethics and legal matters.
- Refer to the CMA's or AMA's Code of Ethics.
- Consider finding and attending an ethics seminar, workshop, or refresher course offered by university continuing medical education programs.
- Call the National Reference Center for Bioethics Literature at Georgetown University (1-800-MED ETHX) for reference help.

HIPPOCRATIC OATH[10]

I swear by Apollo, the physician ... that according to my ability and judgment, I will keep this oath and stipulation: to reckon him who taught me this art equally dear to me as my parents, to share my substance with him and relieve his necessities if required; to regard his offspring as on the same footing with my own brothers, and to teach them this art if they should wish to earn it, without fee or stipulation, and that by precept, lecture and every other mode of instruction ...

I will follow that method of treatment which, according to my ability and judgment, I consider for the benefit of my patients, and abstain from whatever is deleterious and mischievous. I will give no deadly medicine to anyone if asked, nor suggest any such counsel; furthermore, I will not give to a woman an instrument to produce an abortion.

> With the purity and holiness I will pass my life and practice my art. I will not cut a person who is suffering with a stone, but will leave this to be done by practitioners of this work. Into whatever houses I enter I will go unto them for the benefit of the sick and will abstain from every voluntary act of mischief and corruption; and further from the seduction of females or males, bond or free.
>
> Whatever, in connection with my professional practice or not in connection with it, I may see or hear in the lives of men, which ought not be spoken abroad, I will not divulge ...
>
> Hippocrates, 5th century B.C.

LEGAL CONSIDERATIONS

Although ethically sensitive residents and effective communicators are less likely to be sued successfully, there are, nonetheless, several measures they can take to protect themselves from legal action. Here are a list of the most common allegations leading to medical malpractice suits and strategies for avoiding them:

1. Failure to diagnose or treat
2. Failure to obtain appropriate consultation
3. Improper or inaccurate communication among health-care workers
4. Unnecessary, improper, or negligent intervention or treatment
5. Failure to respond to patient inquiry or emergent request
6. Untimely or premature discharge from hospital
7. Failure to obtain legal consent (i.e., prior to anaesthesia)
8. Equipment malfunction
9. Abandonment or discharge from care without arranging appropriate follow-up or referral

Avoiding Litigation

- Avoid coercion, misrepresentation of facts, or leaving conflicts unresolved with patients. Address a patient's dissatisfaction openly and calmly (see chapter 5). Physicians with good communication skills and good relationships with their patients are rarely sued, even if they have made an error in judgment.
- If in doubt about diagnosis, treatment, or procedures in a particular

patient's care, always obtain support for your decision from the senior resident, the attending physician, or a consultant. Document this information in the chart. Your residency malpractice insurance or union (housestaff association) guidelines may require you to discuss all aspects of care with your attending physician, but it is particularly important to record this information when discharging patients. Such guidelines may also come from your program and local licensing authority.

- Document all 'transfers of care' – that is, when signing over post-call, post-shift, or on leaving rotations. Call your hospital's director of professional services, residency director, union representative, or union lawyer if inadequate supervision or co-coverage is available to you during call or emergency-department duty, and document this exchange.

- If you make an error in an order, treatment, or procedure, do not attempt to hide it. Discuss it directly with the senior resident or attending physician to learn how and when the information should be divulged to the patient and family.

- Be sure to obtain proper consent from a patient before a procedure or treatment is started. If you do not, you could be charged with assault and battery. Because the attending physician ultimately is responsible for consent if he or she performs the surgery, determine what information he or she wants given and how it should be given.

- Do not release any information to a third party without documented consent. Ask the hospital's legal department under what circumstances patients have the right to see their own charts. (Usually a physician must be present to explain the aspects of care detailed in the chart.)

- Always double-check the orders of juniors and medical students before signing them, because you are responsible for the consequences.

- Verify how much your attending physician expects to be involved in patient care and decision making and the kind and frequency of documentation expected from you (e.g., once a week in a rehabilitation setting versus several times a day in an intensive-care unit).

- Make sure you have adequate malpractice protection that covers you for the full period of the statute of limitations (the designated number of years a patient can sue a physician after the particular intervention) in your province or state. Investigate whether you are covered for moonlighting rather than assuming you are insured outside the hospital.

- When preparing written prescriptions, *print* drug names, indications, dosing, and timing instructions. Avoid abbreviations, sloppy handwriting, and vague directions like 'prn.' When handing a prescription in, spell the patient's name and the drug name[10] carefully. Avoid oral ('verbal') orders, as they put you, patients, and nursing staff at risk. The AMA House of Delegates, in its 1994 annual meeting, stressed that 'medication errors expose patients to additional but preventable risks leading frequently to prolongation of hospital stay and in some cases contributing to morbidity and mortality, medication errors being the most common case of non-op adverse events (19.4%) and the second most prevalent and second most costly reason for medical malpractice litigation.'
- Maintain good rapport with patients. Avoid making inappropriate or angry comments. Improve cultural sensitivity around ethnic groups.
- Obtain a patient's permission before discussing his or her care with family members.
- Discuss the benefits, risks, and statistical results of a particular procedure/treatment with your patient, and document the discussion in the chart.
- Date and time all patient visits/orders/interventions.
- Always record drug contraindications or allergies, or previous drug interactions.
- Keep your charting and dictations up-to-date.
- Do not agree to partake in research protocols unless they have been cleared by university/hospital ethics committees.
- Verify hospital and local guidelines on curatorship, commitment, use of restraints, and consent issues. Learn whether the age of majority differs from the age of consent to treatment. When a patient is a legal minor, try to have the patient's consent to notify his or her parents. If the treatment is potentially controversial, you may have to obtain parental or guardian consent yourself. Consider obtaining an external consultation.
- Have controversial and sensitive procedures witnessed (e.g., pelvic exams and procedures such as lumbar puncture post-trauma that may result in complications).
- Be aware of legally sensitive areas such as rape, child abuse, custody, and potentially violent behaviour when interviewing patients. Review reporting protocols and make sure you prepare very precise documentation because you may have to give evidence in court.

- Request periodic lectures from your hospital's legal department on specific topics that apply not only to residency, but also to eventual hospital or community-based practice.
- Use caution in e-mailing patients, as confidentiality may be at risk.

Residents may sometimes be asked to testify about patients they have seen, treated, or assessed. Here are several tips for testifying.[11]

- In Canada, call the Canadian Medical Protective Association for guidelines if you are a member. In the United States, speak to your housestaff representative, hospital risk manager, or malpractice insurer.
- Determine whether it would be more appropriate for your attending physician to appear as the person finally responsible for the patient's care.
- Clarify details of your expected appearance (fees, date, time, and location) with the lawyer who has consulted you.
- To avoid wasted time, request that you be called just before your appearance in court and ask whether a detailed written report would be adequate instead of an appearance.
- Discuss with the lawyer who requests your testimony what evidence is expected from you and how to address the judge. Let him or her know if you have objections to the usual procedure of swearing in witnesses with the Christian Bible.
- Bring copies of reports, x-rays, and other documents, because the originals may be kept as evidence. Be prepared with a brief summary or notes.
- Be prepared to state your credentials; you must establish your credibility and expect to be challenged.
- Stay calm and present a serious demeanour. Do not become angry, irreverent, or comical. Use simple terms and do not bluff if you do not know the answer to a question.
- See the resources at the end of this chapter for useful references on coping with the severe stresses of litigation.

OATH FOR NEW DOCTORS[12]

I swear to fulfill, to the best of my ability and judgment, this
   covenant:
I will respect the hard-won scientific gains of those physicians in

whose steps I walk, and gladly share such knowledge as is mine with those who are to follow.

I will apply, for the benefit of the sick, all measures which are required, avoiding those twin traps of overtreatment and therapeutic nihilism.

I will remember that there is art to medicine as well as science, and that warmth, sympathy and understanding may outweigh the surgeon's knife or the chemist's drug.

I will not be ashamed to say 'I know not,' nor will I fail to call in my colleagues when the skills of another are needed for a patient's recovery.

I will respect the privacy of my patients, for their problems are not disclosed to me that the world may know. Most especially must I tread with care in matters of life and death. If it is given me to save a life, all thanks. But it may also be within my power to take a life; this awesome responsibility must be faced with great humbleness and awareness of my own frailty. Above all, I must not play at God.

I will remember that I do not treat a fever chart, or a cancerous growth, but a sick human being, whose illness may affect his family and his economic stability. My responsibility includes these related problems, if I am to care adequately for the sick.

I will prevent disease whenever I can, for prevention is preferable to cure. I will remember that I remain a member of society, with social obligations to all my fellow men, those sound of mind and body, as well as the infirm ...

Louis Lasagna, 1964

REFERENCES

1 Jacobson JA, Tolle SW, Stocking C: Internal medicine residents' preferences regarding medical ethics education. *Acad Med* 1989; 64: 760–764

2 Shreves JG, Moss AH: Residents' ethical disagreements with attending physicians: an unrecognized problem. *Acad Med* 1996; 71(10): 1103–1105

3 Perkins HS: Teaching medical ethics during residency. *Acad Med* 1989; 64: 262–266

4 Jonsen AR, Siegler M, Winslade WJ: *Clinical Ethics*, 4th ed. Macmillan, New York, 1998
5 Beauchamp TL, McCullough LB: *Medical Ethics: The Moral Responsiblities of Physicians*. Prentice-Hall, Englewood Cliffs, NJ 1984
6 Evans KG: *A Medico-Legal Handbook for Canadian Physicians*, 4th ed. Can Med Protect Assoc, Ottawa, 1997
7 Evans KG, Brown NF: *Consent: A Guide for Canadian Physicians*, 3rd ed. Can Med Protect Assoc, Ottawa, 1989
8 Evans KG: *Summary of Federal Legislation and Laws Enacted in the Province of Quebec*. Can Med Protect Assoc, Ottawa, 1990
9 Hutchison R: Do not resuscitate – the writing of no-code orders. *Humane Med* 1990; 6: 135–137
10 *Code of Ethics*. Can Med Assoc, Ottawa, 1997
11 Emson H: Testifying. Courtroom etiquette. Here come the judge – are you ready? *Curr Ther* (*Med Post* suppl) Sept 1989; 25–27
12 Oath for new doctors. *New York Times*, 15 May 1990

OTHER RESOURCES/REFERENCES

Anonymous: *Litigation Assistance: A Guide for the Defendant Physician. Workbook Doc*. American College of Obstetrics and Gynecology, 1986
Benedict MA, O'Rouke KD: *Ethics of Healthcare: An Introductory Textbook*. Georgetown Univ Pr, Washington, 2002
Charles SC: The psychological trauma of a medical malpractice suit: a practical guide. *Am Coll Surg Bull* 1991; 76: 22–26
The *Hastings Center Report* (journal). See also www.thehastingscenter.org

Websites

University of Washington School of Medicine, Bioethics Resources: eduserv.hscer.washington.edu/bioethics/resource/index.html
Kennedy Institute of Ethics: www.georgetown.edu/research/nrcbl
University of British Columbia Library, Bioethicsline: toby.library.ubc.ca/resources/infopage.cfm?id=263

8. Finances

The complete details of budgeting and investing and of planning and setting up a practice are beyond the scope of this chapter. In Canada, more information can be obtained from the CMA and the MD Management Limited network. This network also offers superb tax, financial set-up, and financial counselling seminars, preferred loans, and other services to Canadian residents in training. In the United States, the AMA offers some practice-related workshops,[1] and further financial information can be obtained from unions like the CIR, and occasionally at the hospital or program level. The addresses and telephone numbers of all four organizations are listed in chapter 10.

This chapter touches briefly on the following areas: budgeting, education debts, moonlighting and its tax implications, insurance, obtaining loans, and getting help from other professionals.

BUDGETING

A monthly budget should include the following items:

Income sources
- salary: own and spouse's
- pensions
- bonuses
- investments: dividends, interest, rent
- research or other grants
- alimony
- child support
- moonlighting
- other income

Fixed expenses
- housing: mortgage, rent
- utilities: phone, heat, water, electricity
- property: taxes, maintenance costs
- health care: medical insurance and deductions, medications, dental care
- family coverage
- loan pay-back (e.g., on student loans)
- insurance: life, disability, health, malpractice
- income tax
- transportation: public versus own vehicle (insurance, maintenance, licensing, parking)
- child care
- licensing, professional, and medical society fees
- other expenses

Variable expenses (areas to control)
- retirement investment
- other loans (car, personal, credit cards, line of credit)
- food
- household expenses
- clothing, laundry, cleaning
- pocket money
- transportation
- vacations
- gifts
- charities
- repairs (household)
- entertainment (concerts, films, clubs, television, publications)

CALCULATING YOUR NET WORTH

Assets

Cash or equivalent
Bank accounts, savings	$ _____
Bank accounts, chequing	_____
Life insurance cash value	_____
Other	_____

Securities
  Stocks, common and preferred $ _____
  Mutual funds   _____
  Bonds   _____
  Other   _____

Real estate
  Home $ _____
  Cottage   _____
  Other buildings   _____
  Land   _____
  Other   _____

Other investments
  Medical practice $ _____
  Retirement savings plan   _____
  Home ownership savings plan   _____
  Other business ventures   _____

Other property
  Home furnishings (appliances, furniture) $ _____
  Cars   _____
  Boats, planes, recreational equipment   _____
  Jewellery, furs   _____
  Collections (art, stamps, etc.)   _____
  Other   _____

Debts owed to you $ _____

Miscellaneous $ _____

  Total assets $ _____

Liabilities

Mortgages outstanding
  Home $ _____
  Other buildings   _____
  Land   _____
  Other   _____

Loans outstanding
  Banks, savings and loan $ _____

Broker	$ _____
Insurance policy loan	_____
Other (student)	_____
Other	_____
Taxes	
Income tax (federal and provincial/state)	$ _____
Property	_____
Other	_____
Bills outstanding	$ _____
Miscellaneous	$ _____
Total liabilities	$ _____

Net Worth (assets minus liabilities)

EDUCATION DEBTS

Most provinces in Canada allow a six-month grace period after completion of medical school before charging interest on government loans, but there is some variation. In Quebec, for instance, the grace period is often allowed to continue through residency, which is classified as postgraduate education. Check these regulations with your university's registrar, postgraduate medical office, or an accountant familiar with residents' issues.

Education debts can be a source of extreme stress for residents in the United States, where loans have a two-year interest-deferment period during internship and a ten-year payback limit after completion of medical school. Since residency lasts from four to six years, these conditions can be a source of considerable stress. Residents can request a forbearance to not make payments during residency, but interest charges will generally start after the two-year period. (AMSA, the CIR, and the American Medical Association are lobbying to change the legislation governing these conditions. For updates see the Resident Resource section of the AMA website, www.ama-assn.org, or call 1-866-737-2979. You can also check with the Federal Student Aid Information Center (U.S.) at 1-800-4 FED AID.)

MEDICAL MOONLIGHTING AND ITS TAX IMPLICATIONS

Moonlighting can provide a lucrative source of added income, but the following factors should be weighed:

- whether the residency program policies approve of moonlighting. Be aware that some programs will undermine your attempts at lobbying to limit residency hours by pointing out that residents voluntarily seek out extra (moonlighting) hours.
- provincial or state restrictions on moonlighting (e.g., hospital versus outpatient settings, applicable hours). The ACGME, for instance, prohibits work within one period of a regular residency-scheduled shift.
- whether your malpractice insurance provides coverage outside the hospital and whether the moonlighting establishment will offer such coverage
- the need for and availability of supervision
- potential scheduling conflicts with residency and home life
- licensing regulations (i.e., your eligibility to prescribe drugs outside of a training milieu)
- earnings from fees (your employer will deduct a percentage for overhead from your billing, the rates usually ranging from 25 to 40 per cent)
- get the overhead rate stated in writing and signed by an authorized official
- keep a record of your billings and ask your employer for official receipts
- availability of support, secretarial services, and referral sources

Self-Employed Physicians

Moonlighting will allow you to increase tax deductions and credits because you are a self-employed physician. These can include:

- rent and administration charges
- salaries and employee benefits
- medical supplies
- office taxes and insurance
- office supplies and expenses
- office telephones and other equipment
- medical journals, textbooks
- office repairs and maintenance
- all other expenses that help you earn income (e.g., cleaning bills)
- convention expenses

- continuing expenses
- entertainment expenses
- malpractice insurance
- professional services
- travelling expenses (a percentage of your car expenses related to your practice)
- office at home
- interest and bank charges; any interest that you must pay on loans used for business purposes or for earning income and any bank charges related to these loans
- leasing fees (automobile/equipment)
- depreciation of furniture and textbooks
- moving expenses to relocate after residency

OTHER TAX DEDUCTIONS

Your accountant will advise you as to how purchasing government bonds, and pension and retirement investment plans (i.e., Registered Retirement Savings Plans in Canada, and Individual Retirement Accounts in the United States), can reduce your tax load.

If you are not moonlighting (i.e., not self-employed), your tax deductions and credits may be limited to the following: tuition, monthly student deduction, equipment and textbooks, exam and insurance fees, and moving expenses (in the first year of residency), besides the standard deductions and credits detailed on tax forms.

Other tax areas to explore with your accountant depend on your particular circumstances and include child care, interest on mortgages (in the United States), investment losses, medical expenses (in excess of a certain percentage of your income), charitable or political donations, sales tax credits, child education plans, and spousal income sharing.

INSURANCE

Make sure you explore and fully consider all insurance options. Check your housestaff agreement for details.

Life Insurance Terms and Definitions

- *Whole life*: provides a fixed amount of insurance protection and an accumulation of savings in exchange for a regular premium until the insured's death.

- *Limited payment life*: whole life insurance for which the premiums are level but paid over a specified period (e.g., 20-pay life, single-premium life)
- *Endowment policies*: combines life insurance and savings as in whole life; however, the policy has a specified maturity date. If the policy holder lives to this maturity date, he or she can opt to receive the face value as a lump sum or to receive payments for life or over a specified number of years.
- *Participating*: policy holders are given a share in the total profitability of the insuring company. This is commonly called a dividend, but is in reality a refund on premium overpayments.
- *Non-participating*: policy holders have no rights to share in the profits of the company. The premium is fixed and is calculated on the basis of an estimate of interest rates, administration costs, and future mortality.
- *Double indemnity*: the beneficiary receives twice the face value of the policy if the insured's death is the result of an accident.
- *Term (or temporary) insurance*: called 'pure protection' because it has no cash-surrender or loan value. Policies are insured for specified periods, and benefits are paid only if death occurs within the term of the policy.
- *Level term*: the face value remains constant over the life of the policy.
- *Decreasing term*: the face value of the policy decreases each year, but the premium remains the same.
- *Renewable term*: can be renewed after a prescribed period of time.
- *Convertible term*: may be converted to permanent coverage within a prescribed period without evidence of insurability.

Most residents in Canada and the United States are provided a combination of life, health, and disability insurance through their hospitals, housestaff unions, or university. Ask your hospital resident representative about your coverage, and if none is available contact your provincial or state medical association about available programs.

BUYING LIFE INSURANCE

- Look for the lowest-cost renewable term insurance available.
- Do not be dazzled by the projections of 'cash value' accumulations. These are usually based on assumptions favourable to the company.

- Whole life insurance is expensive and very rarely makes financial sense.
- Provincial and state medical association group plans may provide term insurance at one-half to one-fifth the cost of similar individual policies.
- Ask your association representative to comment on any deficiencies or agent claims existing in the group policy.
- Discuss your life insurance needs with the provincial or state medical association's insurance adviser to see what coverage (if any) you need. Many single physicians starting out in practice need none at all or just enough to cover their debts. Once they marry and have a family, their needs change. You should reassess your needs annually to cover any changes in your lifestyle.
- Even though they do not need any life insurance coverage, some physicians obtain the minimum unit amount from their local medical association to protect their future insurability. Failure to do so would jeopardize their ability to obtain future coverage if a medical problem develops.

Disability Insurance

Discuss your disability insurance needs with your provincial or state association's insurance adviser to determine whether you are adequately covered. You may be covered by the hospital for a portion of your income, but you might want to supplement this with an additional amount before starting out in practice. When you begin practice, estimate your expected income over the first two years and obtain the appropriate amount of disability coverage. As your income increases, your coverage can increase until it reaches the maximum allowed. Initially you may elect a low qualification period (e.g., fourteen days) before receiving payments, but as your finances become more stable you can increase the length of this period and reduce the cost of premiums.

Compare your medical association's disability plan with those of private companies. You may find that some of these companies will not sell insurance coverage if you participate in your medical association's plan. Physicians who want more coverage than the association plan allows buy some coverage from a private company before buying more from the association. Before buying such a policy, however, ask your provincial association to review the private company's proposal. Your choice will depend on your annual earnings and the amount of protection you want. See the insurance agent of the medical association annually to reassess your needs.

Buying Disability Insurance

- Check with your hospital representative to see whether you are already covered.
- Buy the insurance while you are healthy; you will not usually qualify after you become disabled.
- You may want to supplement your present coverage through your medical association policy or a private plan.
- Medical association plans may be 30 to 60 per cent cheaper than private plans.
- Be wary of agents' scare tactics and 'smoke and mirror' tactics.
- Select a short 'elimination period' until your finances are well established.
- Premiums are neither tax-deductible nor creditable, but benefits are not taxable.
- Ask your medical association's representative to comment on any deficiencies a private agent claims exist in the group policy.

Malpractice Insurance

In Canada, one body – the CMPA, a mutual medical defence organization – provides professional liability protection to its members. In the United States, details of malpractice coverage should be explored through state medical associations or the hospital or moonlighting establishment for which you are working.

Other Insurance

Risk management, automobile, and homeowner's insurance are further options to be explored with your broker.

OBTAINING A LOAN / LINE OF CREDIT

- Banks are in business to make money from lending. They are not lending you money as a favour. Shop around!
- Be businesslike when dealing with your banker; see him or her by

appointment and prepare complete and accurate documentation. You may want to suggest in the interview that you might want to do all your banking (personal and professional) at one branch if the deal is favourable.

- Ask for the prime rate plus ¼ per cent on loans with variable interest rates. Make the banker justify any higher rate.
- A fair rate to expect is prime + ½ per cent to prime + 1½ per cent for a variable rate. A fixed rate is more expensive but may be useful if you expect interest rates to rise.
- Establish a line of credit upon which you can draw during the first six months so that you pay interest only on the funds you use.
- Through MD Management Limited, the Canadian Medical Association helps physicians who are setting up a practice to obtain loans at preferred rates. Various U.S. banks such as Citibank do so as well. Check with your union or medical association representative for details.

HELP FROM OTHER PROFESSIONALS

Residents need help from other professionals, especially as they finish training and consider starting up a practice. Obtain references from your state/provincial medical association or from colleagues. The CIR also provides such information.

What a Good Accountant / Financial Planner Can Do for You

- set up a record-keeping system for your practice when you start
- provide you with monthly and formal financial statements that will summarize the financial health of your practice
- help you budget and plan for the post-residency period
- prepare income tax returns (some local medical associations offer income tax preparation services for residents at a reduced rate)
- advise on financial investments
- discuss retirement, estate, and tax planning

Choosing an Accountant

The ideal accountant should have the following:

- experience with a medical practice
- ability to communicate in a clear, concise, and professional manner
- ability to provide responsible leadership for your financial affairs

Other Considerations

- Once the accountant sets up a bookkeeping system, make sure you have a good understanding of how it works.
- Ensure that the system is being maintained properly so that you are not paying the accountant for jobs that your aide could do.
- Take your accountant with you when you consult with other financial advisers or grant permission for them to communicate. He or she will have a good understanding of your financial affairs and will be able to interpret the advice and its implications.

What a Good Lawyer Can Do for You

Ask the housestaff union for the name of the lawyer it retains to assist residents, usually free of charge, for matters related to residency (e.g., contract abuses). A good lawyer can also provide the following:

- draw up formal contracts between you and your co-workers when you start practice
- advise on lease agreements, mortgages, deeds, by-laws, and so on about the location of your practice
- advise on personal matters such as wills
- advise on investments, taxes, and so forth

Important Considerations in Dealing with a Lawyer

- Avoid choosing a friend as a business lawyer, as it may be awkward to change lawyers later.
- Ask your family lawyer, colleagues, or accountant to recommend a business lawyer.
- Ensure that the lawyer can communicate with you in a manner you can understand.
- Make the most of the time spent with the lawyer by making sure that your material is organized and that you are providing all the information he or she needs to do the job well.

POST-RESIDENCY HELP

What a Stockbroker Can Do for You

- look after/buy-and-sell transactions
- provide prompt, accurate execution of orders
- provide a record of your holdings

- make reliable market forecasts
- provide timely technical and fundamental research
- give insight into your investment needs

What a Real Estate Agent Can Do for You

- show you what is available for purchase and give expert appraisals
- help you choose the best location for your office
- help arrange details of leases
- advise you on investment property
- refer you to another agent on matters that are outside his or her area of expertise

What a Good Business Management Consultant Can Do for You

- offer expertise and problem solving on various aspects of the practice such as collections, income distribution, and partnership terms; help set up a medical practice, including choosing a good location, training staff, and so on
- help you prioritize financial costs (home purchase, debt payment, forming investment/credit strategies, etc.)
- provide practice surveys and business analysis
- give specialized consultation on financial investments, personal and family budgeting, and so forth

Risk management, automobile, and homeowner's insurance are further options to be explored with your broker.

REFERENCES

1 *Guide to Establishing a Medical Practice.* MD Management Ltd, Ottawa, 1990 (Much of this chapter is reprinted with permission from this guide.)

OTHER SOURCES

For information on AMA Practice Management Workshops for Residents, see www.ama-assn.org/ama/pub/category/8921.html

McDougall B, Reardon, M: *The Complete Idiot's Guide to Personal Finance for Canadians.* Alpha/Prentice-Hall, Scarborough, ON, 2002 (U.S. equivalents of this guide are available.)

9. Thoughts on the End of Residency

In Greek mythology, Procrustes was a robber who pretended to be an innkeeper on the road to Athens. Travellers seeking success in that city would stop at the inn, where Procrustes would tie them to a bed and adjust them to its length, cutting off the limbs of those who were too tall and stretching those who were too short. He was eventually killed by the hero Theseus.

Residency is truly a modern 'Procrustean voyage,' where conformity, even to deforming principles, can be the price of success. Musical, creative, playful, spontaneous, even romantic aspects of our lives may be cut off if we're not careful. There is no modern-day Theseus to intervene to preserve our integrity, to remind us of our need to remain whole. Our superiors and patients often expect too much of us.

Postgraduate medical education can be a time of great personal growth as well as stress and doubt. The completion of residency marks a departure from the many years of study and training and a shift towards independence and autonomy, away from attending physicians, senior residents, and the hospital hierarchy. Choices have to be made about fellowships, subspecialties, private versus hospital practice, urban versus rural practice, and moves to new locations. Priorities have to be re-examined in the light of having more free time after years of living in an externally imposed structure. Debts wait unpaid. Residents often feel emotionally numb at the end of their training, wondering if they will be able to maintain competence and empathy. They also experience mixed feelings of nostalgia or even loss over 'moving on,' and of pride and accomplishment, tinged with panic, in having become full-fledged physicians.

Various factors can make starting a practice unnerving. Many patients have unrealistic expectations about their health and of their physicians, resulting in a marked increase in litigation against physicians. Malpractice claims in North America have more than doubled over the last ten years. In Canada, patients may consult an excessive number of physicians because health care is perceived to be 'free of charge.' At the same time, provincial programs are being cut, hospitals closed, and the job mobility of new physicians curtailed. In the United States, many patients and some physicians have come to see their exchange as being based on profit and consumerism, and overseen by corporate insurance or managed-care companies that dictate policy and, indeed, what is to be considered acceptable treatment. In both countries constantly advancing technology sometimes humiliates patients and increasingly removes physicians from the bedside. Continuity of care is lost. Overall, physicians find their decision-making power diminished or diluted. These developments and others, including slashed health-care budgets, forced hospital mergers, and concerns about autonomy and wages, significantly reduce job satisfaction.

The media present a worrying image of the physician–patient relationship. Back in 1989 *Time* magazine reported the results of a poll in the United States.[1] A large proportion of patients believed that physicians have no real interest in them, that only one in two 'explains things well enough,' and that physicians' prestige had declined over the previous ten years. *Time* concluded, 'Never have doctors been able to do so much for their patients and rarely have patients seemed so ungrateful.' A survey conducted in 2001 by the Association of American Medical Colleges[2] demonstrated that the majority of graduating medical students that year agreed that changes in the health-care system had impaired physicians' independence. These students also believed that medicine would become less financially rewarding, that administrative and legal liabilities were increasingly burdensome, that a medical career interrupted family life too much and that physicians will be even less respected over time. Finally – perhaps a final blow – a physician shortage is predicted in both the United States and Canada, and this implies a greater workload.[3]

Despite these trends, there are reasons to remain optimistic about the future of residency training and medicine in general in North America. New fields are flourishing, from psycho-immunology to genetic engineering to narrative medicine, new cures are pending, and there is an ever-growing emphasis on prevention. Exciting new technologies, like telemedicine and cyber-surgery links to underserved communities, and an ever-expanding medical Internet are gaining new applications. A growing holistic movement with proponents such as Andrew Weil, MD, and Jon Kabat-Zinn, MD, have emphasized the mind–body connection and how the physician–patient relationship has its own capacity to heal. Best of all, doctors are insisting on taking better care of themselves and are spending more time with their loved ones, and this makes them better physicians and happier human beings.

OPTIONS AFTER RESIDENCY

The Fellowship Option

Setting up practice is only one choice available to graduating residents. Other options include Master's or Doctorate degrees in medical ethics, business/management, humanities, education, or epidemiology. Fellowships, which last from one to three years fall into three categories: clinical, research, or combined.

A fellowship can provide an opportunity to develop a subspecialty, publish, and enhance the possibilities of an academic appointment. (In some university centres a fellowship, with resultant publications, is required before an academic appointment is granted.) It may allow you to sample a new university setting or city, postpone setting up practice, and clarify career plans. Discuss these issues with your mentor, residency director, or university fellowship officer. Matters to consider in negotiating a fellowship are similar to those in residency selection and include the following:

- application procedures and interviewing
- selection criteria (e.g., residency completion, provincial or state licensing) and degree of competition
- benefits, funding, and salary (existence of a financial 'ceiling' if one bills for patients seen)
- office space and secretarial services
- teaching, clinical, and call duties
- publication expectations
- assignment of credit or authorship for work done
- possibility of grant renewal or ongoing funding
- obligation to remain with the research department for a stipulated period on completion of the fellowship
- availability or guarantee of a staff position after fellowship

Fellowship Funding

The principal sources of fellowship funding in Canada are the CIHR, Health Canada, and the Natural Sciences and Engineering Research Council.

Current information on most fellowships available in the United States appears in the education issue that the *Journal of the American Medical Association* publishes every August. The number of subspecialty positions has actually been increasing in the United States over the last several years. *Index Medicus* has a listing of articles discussing pertinent issues relating to fellowships (administrative, pedagogic, and so on). It may be worthwhile doing a current-literature search on your area of interest. The AMA-FREIDA program (see chapter 10) also has a fellowship data bank.

The fellowship office at the university at which you hope to train can provide information on deadlines, addresses, and application procedures of provincial and state funding bodies. In addition, write to specialty associations, because they often offer funding or scholarships, and their data banks provide information on fellowships in North America. Other potential sources of funding include the following:

- employment under attending physician ('staffman') grants
- hospital research institutes
- residency extension (postgraduate year 5 or 6)
- junior staff appointments
- agencies such as the National Cancer Institute or Heart and Stroke Foundation
- private industry (e.g., pharmaceutical companies)
- self-funded clinical fellowships where one bills for patients seen
- other foundation awards

Academic Medicine

Many graduate specialists emerging from residency or fellowship training choose to embark on full-time university-based academic careers. Guidelines for selecting an academic position include clarifying:

- what academic rank will be offered in the position (i.e., lecturer versus assistant professor), and what mechanisms permit promotion
- whether tenure will be available and how it is granted
- whether cross-appointments with other departments are permitted or encouraged

- What grants or financial resources are held by the department and how your income might be guaranteed
- whether sabbaticals will be available and at what frequency
- what the mission statement of the medical school, hospital, department, and division are, and whether these are compatible with your goals
- how much time will be allocated or protected for research versus clinical service
- details of the research environment: lab personnel, office space, provision of materials and supplies (such as computer software)
- what support (i.e., mentoring) will be available for research start-up
- how much inpatient or outpatient clinical work is expected and what opportunities for teaching will be available
- financial issues such as salaries, billing 'ceilings' (and where surplus money goes when you surpass a ceiling), income split between salary and clinical work, benefits (insurance / leaves of absence), office selection and office staff, moving expense reimbursement
- interview procedures (see chapter 2)

During final negotiations for the academic post, seek a written offer summarizing the above points. Discuss the offer with family, your spouse, friends, and possibly your lawyer, as they will all help you clarify ambiguities in the offer and uncertainties in your own mind.[4]

Locum Tenens

Many graduating residents feel unprepared to settle down in one practice or academic setting. They may wish to work part-time, travel, pay off student loans in a hurry, or explore cities where they might wish to settle eventually. The advantages of locum tenens (Latin for 'place holder') positions include the large variety of practice settings, flexible scheduling, low office overhead, and low start-up fees and living expenses. You can find locums by word of mouth, through medical journals, licensing bodies, state or provincial medical association registries, or your professional specialty association. At least twenty-five medical-placement agencies exist in the United States and Canada. See www.locumtenens.com and www.physicianwork.com.

When negotiating with the placement agency or a specific medical facility, find out the mechanism of payment (hourly/daily, rates or fee for service), overhead percentage deducted from your salary, and whether there is a minimum commitment time. Inquire whether you will be provided with provincial or state licensing, housing, and health and malpractice insurance. Don't be afraid to shop around or to negotiate firmly for benefits.

International/Humanitarian/Volunteer Medicine

Many graduates decide to work part-time in a free, low-cost, or community-based clinic as a way of 'giving something back' and of enhancing skills for 'hands-on, low technology' primary care. Most states and provinces can provide lists of public-health or community clinics. The Red Cross holds health fairs across the United States, and recruits volunteers for health screening programs. Other physicians seek experience abroad in Third World countries. Often contacts can be made through American or Canadian medical schools who have affiliate programs overseas or through agencies such as CUSO, the World Health Organization, and the Pan American Health Organization. Here are some specific resources for medical opportunities abroad:[5]

- The National Council for International Health (NCIH), 1701 K Street, NW, Suite 600, Washington, DC 20006. (202) 833-5900
- Health Volunteers Overseas, c/o Washington Station, P.O. Box 65157, Washington, DC 20035. (202) 296-0928
- International Medical Corps, 12233 West Olympic Blvd, Suite 280, Los Angeles, CA 90064. (310) 826-7800; fax (310) 442-6622
- Doctors of the World, 375 West Broadway, 4th floor, New York, NY 10012. (212) 226-9890
- Doctors Without Borders, 11 East 26th Street, Suite 1904, New York, NY 10010 (212) 679-6800 (telephone/fax). In Canada, see www.msf.ca.

Clinical Practice Options

Trying to decide where and how to set up a practice may prove daunting for the graduating resident. Options include group versus private versus hospital-based settings, salaried versus fee-for-service positions, HMOs, and public- versus private-sector institutions.

A new physician can join an already-established group practice and pay overhead or buy into the partnership. Retiring physicians often sell their practices.

Practice opportunities are usually listed in medical journals and association bulletins or sent to physicians by recruitment agencies ('head hunters'). Information on the geographic distribution of physicians in the United States can be found in an annual AMA publication called *Physician Distribution and Medical Licenses in the United States*. Talk to your medical accountant about all options and financial and contractual obligations before signing on. Consider attending one of the AMA's annual practice management workshops for residents which tour the country. Topics include 'Starting Your Practice' and 'Joining a Partnership or Group Practice.' Information and up-to-date publications can be obtained from the AMA Department of Practice Management at 1-800-366-6968.

In Canada, contact MD Management at 1-613-731-9331 regarding literature, practice workshops, and a list of financial advisers in your city or province familiar with these issues. Provincial medical associations list job openings in urban and rural settings.

For information about rural health placements/possibilities in the United States, see Ricketts TC (ed), *Rural Health in the United States* (Oxford Univ Pr, Oxford, 1991) and check out the following web resources:

- Rural Health Education Partnerships program: www.wvrhep.org
- National Rural Recruitment and Retention Network: www.3rnet.org
- National Health Service Corps: bphc.hrsa.gov/nhsc
- Indian Health Service: www.ihs.gov
- Office of Rural Health Policy: www.ruralhealth.hrsa.gov
- Rural Information Center Health Service: www.nal.usda.gov/ric/richs
- National Rural Health Services Research Database: www.muskie.usm .maine.edu/research/ruralheal
- National Rural Health Association: www.nrharural.org
- Rural Health Policy Research Institute: www.rupri.org

SUMMARY

As you finish your residency, remember that your learning does not stop there.[6] You will require continuing medical education as long as you call yourself a physician. Give yourself permission to explore all of your options: if you tire of clinical practice, you can conduct research, write, broadcast, consult, invent, administer, mediate, and become politically active around medical and other issues. You can join academia and become the kind of professor who humanizes the experience of learning for both students and residents. Your vocation within medicine can change and grow as you do.

Whatever your choice, remember the satisfaction of providing good and ethical care, of making accurate diagnoses, of helping someone feel better and regain a sense of dignity in the face of illness. Remember the honour of knowing what your patients have told you and no one else, and of being present at the key moments of their birth, life, and dying. Always find that balance between lifestyle and service that our predecessors could not imagine or attain. Physician, heal thyself.

REFERENCES

1 Dolan B, Gwynne SC, Simpson JC: Sick and tired: uneasy patients may be surprised to find their doctors are worried too. *Time* 31 July 1989; 28–33
2 AAMC 2000 Graduate Questionnaire, cited in *The New Physician*, May/June 2001; 4
3 Cooper RA: Economic and demographic trends signal an impending physician shortage. *Health AFF* (Millwood) 2002; 21: 140–154
4 Fuerst M: US council revises work regulations of residents. *Med Post* 3 Apr 1990; 22
5 Fox RD, Mazmanian PE, Putnam RW: *Changing and Learning in the Lives of Physicians*. Praeger, New York, 1989
6 Peterkin AD: From socks to souls: how will I manage? *Curr Ther* (*Med Post* suppl) Dec 1988; 6

OTHER RESOURCES

Gold BD, Haslam RHA, Tallett S, Feldman W: On seeking a career in academic medicine, or how to go about getting a job. *CRMCC* 1995; 28(5): 288
Werner D, Thurnam C: *Where There Is No Doctor*. Hesperian Foundation, Berkeley, CA, 2002. An excellent primer on working in under-serviced Third World settings
Nichols M: At the breaking point: doctors and nurses rethink their careers. *Maclean's Magazine* Jan 2001; 22–32
The Coker Group, Max R: *AMA – Starting a Medical Practice. The Physician's Handbook for Successful Practice Start-Up*. AMA, Chicago, 1996
Daniel L: *Preparing for Medical Practice Made Ridiculously Simple*. MedMaster, Miami, 1998
Professionalism in Medicine – A Discussion Paper. CMA, Ottawa, 2001

Goldman, LS (ed): *The Handbook of Physician Health: The Essential Guide to Under-standing the Health Care Needs of Physicians.* AMA, Chicago, 2000

The Resilient Physician (www.The Resilient Physician.com; 1-888-629-2313) is a bi-monthly newsletter 'dedicated to today's physicians, medical families, and medical organizations' and contains practical tips on improving the quality of life for doctors and their patients.

Conferences

The AMA and the CMA (American Medical Association / Canadian Medical Association) hold an International Conference on Physician Health every two years. Contact either organization for meeting information and ask to be added to their Physician Health e-mail list.

10. Resources

APPLYING FOR RESIDENCY

American Academy of Family Physicians
8880 Ward Parkway
Kansas City, MO 64114
Tel: (800) 274-2237
Fax: (816) 822-0580
http://www.aafp.org

AMA-FREIDA (Fellowship and Residency Electronic Interactive
Database) Computer listing of residencies. Access with data on programs and institutions. American Medical Association and Resident Physician Section (AMA-RPA), 515 North State Street, Chicago IL 60610
Tel (312) 464-5000
http://www.ama-assn.org/ama/pub/category/2997.html

American Medical Student Association
1902 Association Drive
Reston, VA 22091
Tel (703) 620-6600 or (800) 767-2266
fax (703) 620-5873
http://www.amsa.org

Accreditation Council for Graduate Medical Education
515 North State Street, Suite 2000
Chicago, IL 60610

National Resident Matching Program
2510 M Street NW, Suite 201

Washington, DC 20037-1141
http://www.nrmp.org

The Residency Page
http://www.kemc.edu/residency.html

National Center for Evaluation of Residency Programs
http://www.ncerp.com

Educational Commission for Foreign Medical Graduates
3624 Market Street
Philadelphia, PA 19104
Tel: (215) 386-5900
Fax: (215) 387-9963
http://www.ecfmg.org/faimer/ifme/forms/ifmeprt2.pdf

MATCH INFORMATION

Canadian Resident Matching Service
Sandra Banner, Executive Director
802-151 Slater Street
Ottawa, ON K1P 5H3
Tel: (613) 237-0075 or (800) 291-3727
Fax: (613) 563-2860
http://www.carms.ca

The Electronic Residency Application Service
http://www.aamc.org/students/eras/start.htm

National Resident Matching Program
2501 M Street NW, Suite 1
Washington, DC 20037-1307
Tel: (202) 828-0566
http://www.nrmp.org

INTERNET RESOURCES

The Residency Page

http://www.webcom.com/~wooming/residenc.html
This Web site is a list of medical residencies available on the WWW,
maintained by family-practice resident Mike Woo-Ming.

National Center for Evaluation

http://www.ncerp.com
This Web site by the National Center for Evaluation of Residency Programs is an information resource for administrators of residency programs, designed to enhance hospital residency programs.

AAMC Programs

http://www.aamc.org/about/progemph/eras
This Web site is the home page for ERAS (The Electronic Residency Application Service), a service of the Association of American Medical Colleges. ERAS transmits residency applications, letters of recommendation, deans' letters, and transcripts from medical schools to residency program directors using the Internet.

CME Web Sites

American College of Physicians Journal Club
http://www.acponline.org/journals/acpjc/jcmenu.htm

American Medical Association, medical science and education
http://www.ama-assn.org/med-sci/cme.htm

Journal Club on the Web (general medicine)
http://www.webcom.com/mjlijweb/jrnlclb

Journal of Family Practice Journal Club
http://www.jfp.msu.edu/jclub/Indexes/jcindex.htm

Medconnect (CME, cases, teaching files, review courses)
http://www.medconnect.com

Stanford primary care teaching modules
http://www.-med.stanford.edu

Virtual Hospital CME
http://indy.radiology.uowa.edu/Providers/Providers.html

Useful Medical Web Sites

American Medical Association
http://www.ama-assn.org

Canadian Medical Association Online
http://www.cam.ca

College of Family Physicians of Canada
http://www.cfpc.ca

Cyberspace Hospital
http://www.CH.nus.sg

Emergency medicine and primary care
http://www.embbs.com

Hyperdoc, U.S. National Library of Medicine
http://www.nlm.hih.gov

Journal of Family Practice, Journal Club
http://jfp/msu.edu/jclub/jclub.htm

Med Help International (patient information)
http://medhlp.netusa.net

Medical Matrix
http://www.medmatrix.org/index.stm

MEDLINE

http://www.healthgate.com/HealthGate/MEDLINE/
search-advanced.shtml

Medweb electronic newletters and journals
http://www.cc.emory.edu/WHSCL/medweb.html

Multimedia medical reference library
http://www.med-library.com

National Physician Job Listing Directory
http://www.embbs.com/job/jobs.html

Physicians' home page
http://www.silverplatter.com/physicians

Primary Care Internet Guide
http://www.uib.no/isf/guide/family.htm

Society of Teachers of Family Medicine
http://stfm.org

Virtual Hospital
http://indy.radiology.uiowa.edu

Webdoctor
http://www.gretmar.com/webdoctor/home.html

WWW Virtual Medical Library/Cliniweb
http://www.ohsu.edu/cliniweb/wwwvl

Yahoo, Medicine
http://www.hahoo.com/Health/Medicine

Medical Journal Internet Addresses

American Family Physician
http://www.aafp.org/family/afp/index.html

American Journal of Preventive Medicine
http://aaup.pupress.princeton.edu:70/CGI/cgi-bin/hfs.cgi/66/
oxford/ajpm.ctl

Archives of Family Medicine
http://www.ama-assn.org/public/journals/fami/famihome.htm

Archives of Internal Medicine
http://www.ama-assn.org/public/journals/inte/intehome.htm

Archives of Pediatrics and Adolescent Medicine
http://www.ama-assn.org/public/journals/ajdc/ajdchome.htm

British Medical Journal
http://www.bmj.com/bmj

Canadian Family Physician
http://www.cfpc.ca/canadian/htm

Canadian Medical Association Journal
http://www.cma.ca/journals/cmaj/index.html

Digital Journal of Ophthalmology
http://www.cam.ca/journals/cmaj/index.html

Family Practice Newletter
http://www.med.ufl.edu/medinfo/pcnews/pcnews22.html

International Journal of Medicine
http://www.cityscape.co.uk/users/ad88/psych.htm

Journal of Family Practice
http://www.phypc.med.waybne.edu/jfp/jfp.htm

Source: Anthes DL et al: Internet resources for family physicians. *Can Fam Physician* 1997; 43: 1104–1113

Other Web Sites

OSLER/OVID
http://www.cma.ca/osler/index.htm

MEDLINE by Pub Med
http://www.ncbi.nlm.hih.gov/PubMed

Cochrane Library
http://www.updateuse.com/clibpw/clib.htm

Abstracts of Cochrane reviews
http://www.update-software.com/cochrane/cochrane-frame.html

York Systematic Reviews
http://www.york.ac.uk/inst/crd/srinfo.htm

Medical Journals

Canadian Medical Association Journal
http://www.cma.ca/cmaj-f/index.asp

British Medical Journal
http://www.bmj.com

Annals of Internal Medicine
http://www.acponline.org/journals/annals/annaltoc.htm

JAMA
http://jama.ama-assn.org

Lancet
http://www.thelancet.com

Free Medical Journals
http://www.freemedicaljournals.com

Medscape General Medicine
http://www.medscape.com/Medscape/GeneralMedicine/journal/public/mgm.journal.html

Amedeo
http://www.amedeo.com

Jade
http://www.biodigital.org/jade

Journal Clubs

Critique et pratique
http://www.crsfa.ulaval.ca/umf

CFPC Critical Appraisal
http://www.cfpc.ca/CFP/cfpritindex.htm

Info POEMS; *Journal of Family Practice*
http://www.infopoems.com/POEMs/jcindex.htm

ACP Journal Club
http://www.acponline.org/journals/acpjc/jcmenu.htm

Best Evidence (CD-ROM version)
http://www.acponline.org/catalog/electronic/best_evidence.htm

Bandolier
http://www.jr2.ox.ac.uk/Bandolier/index.html

RESIDENTS' HOUSESTAFF ORGANIZATIONS

Canada

Canadian Association of Interns and Residents
161 Slater Street, Suite 412
Ottawa, ON K1P 5H3
Tel: (613) 234-6448
http://www.cair.ca

PAR-BC
900-610 West Broadway
Vancouver, BC V5Z 4C2
Tel: (604) 876-7636
Fax: (604) 876-7690
Toll free: 1-888-877-2722
E-mail: par@netcom.ca
http://www.par-bc.org

PAIRA
460, 8409-112 Street
Edmonton, AB T6G 1K6
Tel: (403) 432-1749
Fax: (403) 432-1778
(403) 236-4841 (Calgary)
E-mail: paira@planet.con.net

PAIRS
Royal University Hospital
103 Hospital Drive
Saskatoon, SA S7N 0W8
Tel/Fax: (306) 655-2134
E-mail: paris@link.ca
http://www.pairs.com

PARIM
Room AD 107, 720 McDermot Avenue
Winnipeg, MB R3E 0T3
Tel: (204) 787-3673
Fax: (204) 787-2692
http://www.parim.org

PAIRO
505 University Avenue, Suite 1402
Toronto, ON M5G 1X4
Tel: (416) 979-1182 or 1-877-979-1183
Fax: (416) 595-9778
E-mail: pairo@pairo.org
http://www.pairo.org

PARI-MP (for Nova Scotia, New Brunswick, and Prince Edward Island)
Room 443, Bethune Building, Victoria General Hospital
QUII Health Sciences Center
1278 Tower Road
Halifax, NS B3H 2Y9
Tel: (902) 473-7861/473-4091
Fax: (902) 473-4451
E-mail: chebb@atcon.com
http://www.oma.org/ins/pariessentials.htm

PAIRN
Student Affairs Office
Room 2713, Memorial University Medical School
Health Sciences Complex
St John's, NF A1B 3V6
Tel: (709) 737-7118
Fax: (709) 737-6680/6746
http://www.med.mun.ca/pgme/pages/pairn.htm

Fédération des Médécins Résidents du Québec
445 Sherbrooke Street West
Montréal, PQ H3A 1B6
Tel: (514) 282-0256
http://www.cnw.ca/releases/March2003/18/c1876.html

United States

CIR (Committee of Interns and Residents)
386 Park Avenue South, Room 1502
New York, NY 10016
Tel: (212) 725-5500
Fax: (212) 779-2413
http://www.cirdocs.org

Specialty Associations

Aerospace Medical Association
320 South Henry Street
Alexandria, VA 22314
http://www.asma.org

American Academy of Allergy, Asthma, and Immunology
611 East Wells Street
Milwaukee, WI 53202
http://www.aaaai.org

American Academy of Child and Adolescent Psychiatry
3615 Wisconsin NW
Washington, DC 20016
http://www.aacap.org

American Academy of Dermatology
930 Meacham Road

Schaumburg, IL 60172-4965
http://www.aad.org

American Academy of Family Physicians
8880 Ward Parkway
Kansas City, MO 64114
http://www.aafp.org

American Academy of Neurology
2221 University Aveune SE, Suite 335
Minneapolis, MN 55414
http://www.aan.com/professionals

American Academy of Ophthalmology
655 Beach Street
San Francisco, CA 94120
http://www.aao.org

American Academy of Orthopedic Surgeons
6300 North River Road
Rosemont, IL 60018-4226
http://www.aaos.org/wordhtml/home2.htm

American Academy of Otolaryngolgy
1 Prince Street
Alexandria, VA 22314
http://www.si.umich.eduu/HCHS/REPOS-NAT/AcadOtol.html

American Academy of Pediatrics
141 Northwest Point Boulevard
Elk Grove Village, IL 60009-0927
http://www.aap.org

American Association of Colleges of Osteopathic Medicine
5550 Friendship Boulevard, Suite 310
Chevy Chase, MD 20815-7231
http://www.aacom.org

American Association of Dental Schools
1625 Massachusetts Avenue NW, Suite 600
Washington, DC 20036
http://www.adea.org/sections/Endodontics/Report.pdf

American Society of Internal Medicine
2011 Pennsylvania Avenue NW, Suite 800

Washington, DC 20006-1808
http://www.acponline.org

American Society of Nephrology
1101 Connecticut Avenue NW
Washington, DC 20036
http://www.asn-online.org/home.asp

American Society of Plastic and Reconstructive Surgeons
444 East Algonquin Road
Arlington Heights, IL 60005
http://www.plasticsurgery.org

American Thoracic Society
1740 Broadway, 14th floor
New York, NY 10019-4371
http://www.thoracic.org

American Urological Association
1120 North Charles Street
Baltimore, MD 21201
http://www.auanet.org

Association of American Medical Colleges
2450 N Street NW
Washington, DC 20037
http://www.aamc.org

College of American Pathologists
325 Waukegan Road
Northfield, IL 60093-2750
http://www.cap.org

Educational Commission for Foreign Medical Graduates
2624 Market Street
Philadelphia, PA 19104
http://www.ecfmg.org

Endocrine Society
4350 East West Highway, Suite 500
Bethesda, MD 20814
http://www.endo-society.org

National Association of Advisors for the Health Professions
P.O. Box 1518

Champaign, IL 61824
http://www.naaph.org

National Dental Association
5506 Connecticut Avenue NW, Suite 24
Washington, DC 20015
http://www.ndaonline.org

National Medical Association
10121th Street NW
Washington, DC 20001
http://www.nmanet.org

Rehabilitation Physicians Association
1101 Vermont Avenue NW, Suite 500
Washington, DC 20005

Society of Critical Care Medicine
8101 East Kaiser Boulevard, Suite 300
Anaheim, CA 92808-2259
http://www.sccm.org

Society of Thoracic Surgeons
401 North Michigan Avenue
Chicago, IL 60611-4267
http://www.sts.org

SPECIALTY BOARD EXAMS

Canada

The Royal College of Physicians and Surgeons of Canada
774 Echo Drive
Ottawa, ON K1S 5N8
Tel: (613) 730-8177
Fax: (613) 730-8833

OTHER EXAMINATIONS

National Board of Medical Examiners
3750 Market Street
Philadelphia, PA 19104
Tel: (215) 590-9500
Fax: (215) 590-9555

LICENSURE

Canada

British Columbia

Registar's Office
1807 West 10th Avenue
Vancouver, BC V6J 2A9
Tel: (604) 733-7758
Fax: (604) 733-3503

Alberta

Registrar, College of Physicians and Surgeons
900 Manulife Place
10180-101 Street
Edmonton, AB T5J 4P8
Tel: (403) 423-4764
Fax: (403) 420-0651

Saskatchewan

College of Physicans and Surgeons of Saskatchewan
211-4th Avenue South
Saskatoon, SK S7K 1N1
Tel: (306) 244-7355
Fax: (306) 244-0090

Manitoba

The Registrar, College of Physicians and Surgeons of Manitoba
494 St James Street
Winnipeg, MB R3G 3J4
Tel: (204) 774-4344
Fax: (204) 774-0750

Ontario

College of Physicians and Surgeons of Ontario
80 College Street
Toronto, ON M5G 2E2
Tel: (416) 967-2600 (400)
Fax: (416) 961-3330

Quebec

Collège des Médecins du Québec
2170 boulevard René-Lévesque Ouest
Montréal, PQ H3H 2T8
Tel: (514) 933-4441
Fax: (514) 933-3112

New Brunswick

Registrar, Medical Council of New Brunswick
1 Hampton Road, Suite 300
Rothesay, NB E2E 5K8
Tel: (506) 849-5050
Fax: (506) 849-5069

Nova Scotia

Provincial Medical Board of Nova Scotia
5248 Morris Street
Halifax, NS B3J 1B4
Tel: (902) 422-5823
Fax: (902) 422-5035

Prince Edward Island

Registrar's Office
The College of Physicians & Surgeons of Prince Edward Island
Polyclinic, 199 Grafton Street
Charlottetown, PEI C1A 1L2
Tel/Fax: (902) 566-3861

Newfoundland

Office of the Registrar, Newfoundland Medical Board
13 Water Street, Unit 6
St John's, NF A1C 1B2
Tel: (709) 726-8546
Fax: (709) 706-4725

Yukon Territories

Registrar
Yukon Medical Practitioners
Box 2703
Whitehorse, YT Y1A 2C6

Licensing information for Canadians interested in training or working in the United States can be found in the *1990 AMA Graduate Medical Education Guide*, AMA Press, Chicago, 1990: Table 2, Appendix C, p. 735. This table lists over forty states which accept LMCC as reciprocal.

United States

Please refer to the July and January issues of the current year of *Journal of the American Medical Association* for the most recent addresses of all U.S. licensing bodies or consult the AMA website.

NATIONAL MEDICAL ASSOCIATIONS

Canadian Medical Association
1867 Alta Vista Drive
Ottawa, ON K1G 3Y6
Tel: (613) 731-9931 or (800) 267-9703
Fax: (613) 731-9013
http://www.cmaj.ca

American Medical Association
515 North State Street
Chicago, IL 60610
Tel: (312) 464-5000
http://www.ama-assn.org

OTHER ORGANIZATIONS

Canada

Addresses and phone numbers of various Canadian associations may be obtained from the Communications Department at the Canadian Medical Association.

Association of Canadian Medical Colleges
774 Echo Drive
Ottawa, ON K1S 5P2
Tel: (613) 730-0687
Fax: (613) 730-1196
http://www.acmc.ca

Canadian Association of General Surgeons
407-55 Queen Street East
Toronto, ON M5C 1R6
Tel: (416) 361-1233
http://cags.medical.org

Canadian Federation of Medical Students
500-505 University Avenue
Toronto, ON M5G 1X4
Tel: (416) 595-9778
http://www.cfms.org/files/cfms_nomination_ad.pdf

Canadian Healthcare Association
17 York Street
Ottawa, ON K1N 9J6
Tel: (613) 241-8005
Fax: (613) 241-5055
http://www.canadian-healthcare.org

Canadian Resident Matching Service
802-151 Slater Street
Ottawa, ON K1P 5H3
Tel: (613) 237-0075
Fax: (613) 563-2860
http://www.carms.ca

Canadian Medical Protective Association
Carling Square, 560 Rochester Street
Ottawa, ON K1S 4M2
Tel: (613) 236-2100

College of Family Physicians of Canada
2630 Skymark Avenue
Mississauga, ON L4W 5A4
Tel: (905) 629-0900 or (800) 387-6197
Fax: (905) 629-0893
http://www.cfpc.ca

Medical Council of Canada
PO Box 8234, Station T
Ottawa, ON K1G 3H7
Tel: (613) 521-6012
Fax: (613) 521-9417
http://www.mcc.ca

Medical Research Council of Canada
Holland Cross Tower B
5th floor, 1600 Scott Street
Ottawa, ON K1A 0W9
Tel: (613) 954-1809
Fax: (613) 954-1802
http://www.nrc-cnrc.gc.ca/~indcan/report1998/english/mrc_e.html

The Royal College of Physicians and Surgeons of Canada
774 Echo Drive
Ottawa, ON K1S 5N8
Tel: (613) 730-8177
Fax: (613) 730-8833
http://rcpsc.medical.org/index.php3?pass=1

United States

Please refer to the July and January issues of the current year of the *Journal of the American Medical Association* for the most recent addresses of hundreds of medical organizations, including:

American Board of Medical Specialties
American College of Physicians
Association of American Medical Colleges
Council of Medical Specialty Societies
National Board of Medical Examiners

International

Pan American Health Organization
525-23rd Street NW
Washington, DC 20037
Tel: (202) 861-3200
Fax: (202) 223-5971

Pan American Medical Association
c/o Frederic C. Fenig, MD
745 5th Avenue, Suite 403
New York, NY 10151
Tel: (212) 753-6033
Fax: (212) 308-6847

World Medical Association
28, Avenue des Alpes
BP 63 F-01212
Ferney-Voltaire, France
Tel: 33-50-40-75-75
Fax: 33-50-40-59-37
http://www.wma.net/e

World Health Organization
Avenue Appla
CH-1211
Geneva 27, SWITZERLAND
Fax: 41-22-7910746
http://www.who.int/en

Commonwealth Medical Association
c/o BMA House, Tavistock Square
London WC1H 9JP
England
Tel: 44 171 383 6095
E-mail: 72242.3544@compuserve.com
http://commedas.org

British Medical Association
Tavistock Square
London WC1H 9JP
England
Fax: 44 171 383 6403
Hotlines for Physician Stress Counselling:
0 645 200169 or 0 171 935 5982
http://www.bma.org.uk/ap.nsf/Content/_Home_Public

SPECIAL INTEREST GROUPS

United States

Please refer to the July and January issues of the current year of the *Journal of the American Medical Association* for the most recent addresses of these and hundreds of other groups of interest and for new annual conference dates.

American Medical Women's Association
Christian Medical and Dental Society
Gay and Lesbian Medical Association
Institute of Religion and Health
National Library of Medicine
American Association of Physicians for Human Rights

FINANCIAL AND BUSINESS RESOURCES

Canada

MD Management Limited
1867 Alta Vista Drive
Ottawa, ON K1G 5W8
Tel: (800) 267-4022
Fax: (613) 526-1352
http://mdm.ca/md/index.asp

United States

Contact the local CIR chapter and the AMA–Resident Physician section re: Practise Management Workshops.

LEGAL RESOURCES

Canada

Canadian Medical Protective Association
PO Box 8225, Station T
Ottawa, ON K1G 3H7
Tel: (613) 725-2000 or (800) 267-6522
Fax: (613) 725-1300
http://www.cmpa-acpm.ca

United States

Contact your local union, housestaff association, AMA chapter, or hospital legal department.

OTHER RESOURCES

Ask your medical librarian about access to the following publications and journals.

- *Academic Medicine* (formerly Journal of Medical Education)
- *ARS MEDICA*
- *Bellevue Literary Review*
- *British Medical Journal*
- *Canadian Medical Association Journal*
- *Journal of the American Medical Association* (has a regular residents' column called 'On Call')
- *The New Physician*

Also:

- Have your name added to the subscription list of the local and national housestaff organization (i.e., CAIR, CIR) newsletter.
- Read your specialty association journals for residents' forum sections. The American Psychiatric Association's *Psychiatric News*, for instance, has a regular residents' column.

Index

QUESTIONNAIRE

This is the third edition of a book designed for generations of residents. Before passing your copy to a junior, please fill out the following questionnaire to help us keep it useful and up to date. Please complete and mail to: University of Toronto Press, 10 St Mary Street, Suite 700, Toronto, Ontario M4Y 2W8. You can also email Dr Peterkin at apeterkin@mtsinai.on.ca.

Age: **Sex:**

Specialty or residency:

Province or state:

Comments on book's content and layout:

Additional suggested coping tips:

Additional suggested references, resources, addresses:

Are you satisfied with your residency training experience?

How did you find out about *Staying Human during Residency Training?*

Other comments:

Date of response: